Backpacking Nevada

From the book...

Mt. Rose and Bronco Creek (Trip 2)

Reach the floor of Galena Creek canyon at 2.3 miles from the trailhead and stand below this scenic gem, where multiple ribbons of water spill picturesquely down dark rock walls. Downstream, an expansive meadow provides a fine foreground view for the massive hulk of Mt. Rose.

Winchell Lake Trail (Trip 8)

You enter East Humboldt Wilderness just before the crossing of South Fork Angel Creek, a tumbling stream that courses thought a verdant swath of foliage and flowers, with the rugged cliffs of Chimney Rock presenting a dramatic backdrop.

Soldier Lakes Basin (Trip 10)

Eventually, the canyon widens, the grade moderates, and the more open terrain allows for fine views of Soldier Peak. The path veers away from the creek for a time until you wander back though a field of waist-high wildflowers, crossing a spring-fed tributary along the way.

Toiyabe Crest Trail (Trip 15)

The broad basin of the upper Reese River spreads out before you. The rolling hills carpeted with silvery-green sagebrush and the seemingly endless sky bring to mind a cowboy country image—the only missing piece is John Wayne astride his stallion.

Mt. Jefferson Loop (Trip 18)

Now the long plateau atop Mt. Jefferson stretches out before you, where desert-alpine vegetation struggles to attain heights of even 3 to 4 inches, and wildflower blooms are short-lived. Awe-inspiring, 360-degree views are commonplace, with mountains from California to Utah visible on clear days.

Table Mountain Traverse (Trip 19)

Mid-June to mid-July is an excellent time to visit, when the flowers are at their peak and plenty of water is in the streams; late September to early October is a grand time to see the aspens at the height of their glory, audibly complemented by the bugling of male elk.

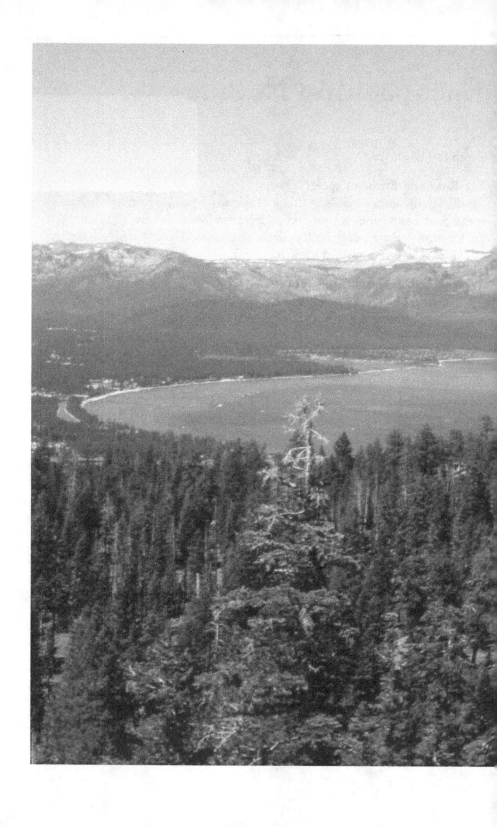

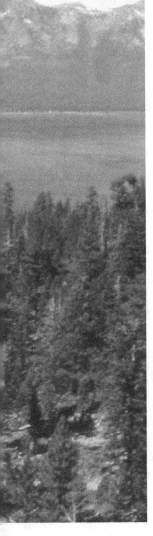

Backpacking
NEVADA

From
Slickrock Canyons
to Granite Summits

Mike White

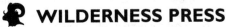

WILDERNESS PRESS
...on the trail since 1967
BERKELEY, CA

Backpacking Nevada: From Slickrock Canyons to Granite Summits

1st EDITION 2004
  2nd printing 2008

Copyright © 2004 by Mike White

Front cover photo copyright © 2004 by Larry Ulrich
Back cover photo copyright © 2004 by Mike White
Interior photos by Mike White
Maps: Mike White
Cover design: Andreas Schueller
Book design: Andreas Schueller and Jaan Hitt

ISBN 978-0-89997-322-7

Manufactured in the United States of America
Distributed by Publishers Group West

Published by: **Wilderness Press**
            1345 8th Street
            Berkeley, CA 94710
            (800) 443-7227; FAX (510) 558-1696
            info@wildernesspress.com
            www.wildernesspress.com
Visit our website for a complete listing of our books and for ordering information.

Cover photos: Cirrus clouds over Ruby Mountains *(front)*;
            Mt. Rose from Slide Mountain—Trip 2 *(back)*
Frontispiece: Lake Tahoe from the Tahoe Rim Trail—Trip 1

SAFETY NOTICE: Although Wilderness Press and the author have made every attempt to ensure that the information in this book is accurate at press time, they are not responsible for any loss, damage, injury, or inconvenience that may occur to anyone while using this book. You are responsible for your own safety and health while in the wilderness. The fact that a trail is described in this book does not mean that it will be safe for you. Be aware that trail conditions can change from day to day. Always check local conditions and know your own limitations.

Dedication

To my wife, my beloved, my helpmate, without whose support and encouragement this book would not exist.

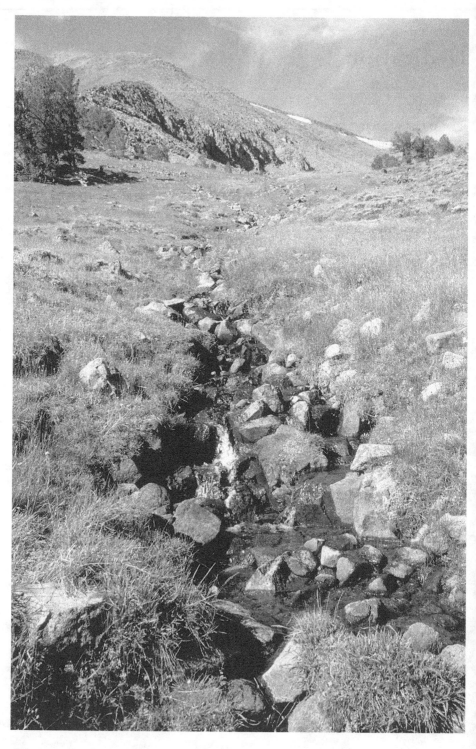

Stream in Bucks Canyon (Trip 18)

Acknowledgments

Over the years many individuals have given their assistance to this project in a variety of ways. First and foremost, my gratitude is extended to Tom Winnett, founder and patriarch of Wilderness Press, who was the first to believe not only in the concept of a guidebook about the backcountry of Nevada, but in my ability to steer that vision into reality. Secondly, Mike Jones, Jannie Dresser, Larry Van Dyke, and the staff at Wilderness Press are due a big thank you for handling this project with their usual diligence and care. Thanks especially to Elaine Merrill and Roslyn Bullas for seeing the project through to completion.

Several friends granted me the privilege of their company on the trail throughout the process of doing the fieldwork, including Dwight Smith, Mike Wilhelm, Dave Peterson, Brian Gervais, John Burton, Keith Catlin, and the youth group from RCF (Leo, Ben, Brian, Danna, Daniel, David, Josh, Karen, Kristen, Peter, Rachel, Steve, and Yun). Their companionship kept my already skewed perspective from getting further out of whack amid so much solitude. Additional thanks are extended to Carmel Bang, Ciera Durling and Mary Ann Williams for helping to make possible so many trips into the Nevada backcountry.

Although this book is already dedicated to my wife, I must thank her again for making this project possible, for without her *Backpacking Nevada* would simply not exist. Her review of the manuscript was much appreciated as well.

Lastly, but most importantly, I thank God for blessing me with the opportunities to enjoy His creation, along with the ability to put together on paper some seemingly coherent thoughts.

—Mike White
March 2004

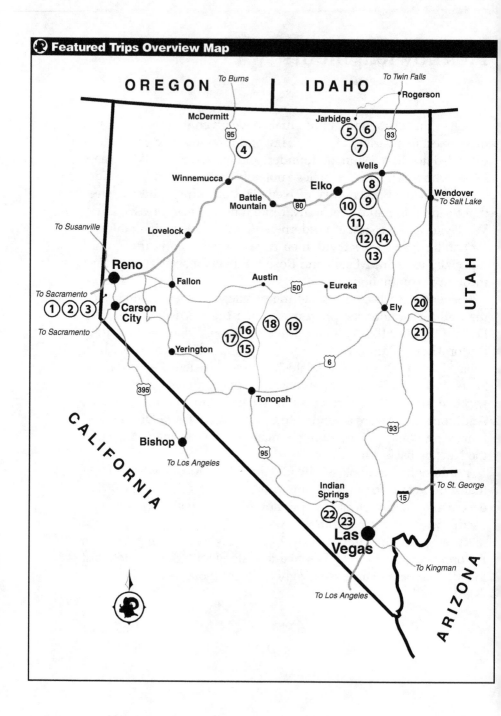

Featured Trips Overview Map

Contents

FEATURED TRIPS OVERVIEW MAP viii

MAP LEGEND xii

FEATURED TRIPS SUMMARY CHART xiii

INTRODUCTION 1
How To Use This Guide 3

GENERAL TIPS ON BACKPACKING IN NEVADA 7

A WORD ABOUT HORSES 11

WILD AREAS OF NEVADA:
Carson Range 15
Santa Rosa Range 16
Jarbidge Mountains 18
East Humboldt Mountains 21
Ruby Mountains 23
Toiyabe Mountains 25
Toquima Range 28
Monitor Range 29
Snake Range 31
Great Basin National Park 32
Spring Mountains 34

FEATURED TRIPS:
Carson Range
    1 Tahoe Rim Trail: Daggett Pass to Brockway Summit 39
    2 Mt. Rose and Bronco Creek 59
    3 Ophir Creek Trail 67
Santa Rosa Range
    4 Summit Trail 75

Jarbidge Mountains

5 Jarbidge and Emerald Lake Loop 85

6 East Fork Jarbidge River and Cougar Creek Loop 93

7 Gods Pocket Peak Trail to Camp Creek 101

East Humboldt Mountains

8 Winchell Lake Trail 107

9 Greys Lake Trail 113

Ruby Mountains

10 Soldier Lakes Basin 119

11 Right Fork Lamoille Creek 125

12 Ruby Lakes 131

13 Ruby Crest Trail 137

14 Overland Lake Trail 155

Toiyabe Mountains

15 Toiyabe Crest Trail 159

16 North Twin and South Twin Rivers Loop 171

17 Stewart Creek Loop 177

Toquima Range

18 Mt. Jefferson Loop 183

Monitor Range

19 Table Mountain Traverse 189

Snake Range

20 Mt. Moriah 195

Great Basin National Park

21 Baker Creek Loop to Baker and Johnson Lakes 203

Spring Mountains

22 Bonanza Trail 211

23 Charleston Peak: North Loop and South Loop Trails 217

BIBLIOGRAPHY AND SUGGESTED READING 225

INDEX 227

ABOUT THE AUTHOR 230

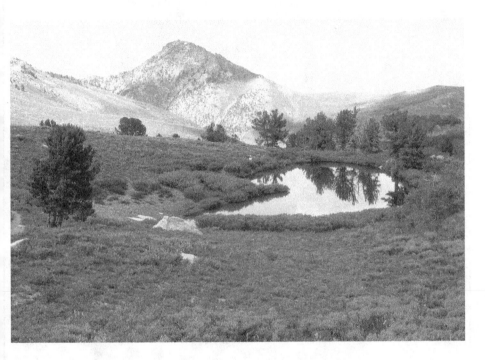

One of the Soldier Lakes with Soldier Peak in the background (Trip 10)

•—— 4.0 ——•	Main Trail with Mileage
- - - - - - - - -	Other Trails
· · · · · · · · · ·	Cross-country Routes
P	Parking
T	Trailhead
————	Road (paved)
— — — — —	Road (gravel or dirt)
– – – – –	Road (4WD)
(80)	Interstate Highway
(50)	U.S. Highway
207	State Highway
(752)	County Road
660	Forest Service Road
⌂	Ranger Station
▲ 10667'	Mountain with Elevation
◯	Lake
～～	Stream
♀	Spring
▲	Campsite

Featured Trips Summary Chart

TRIP	RATINGS (1-10)			DAYS	MILES	ELEVATION GAIN	SHUTTLE MILES
	SCENERY	SOLITUDE	DIFFICULTY				

ually Open:

te May

| 2 Bonanza Trail | 8 | 8 | 8 | 2 | 17 | 5400 | 36 |

d-June

0 Soldier Lakes Basin	8	8	6	2–4	11	2400	N/A
5 Toiyabe Crest Trail	8	10	7	3–5	37	10,250	100
6 North Twin & South Twin Rivers Loop	7	9	6	2	14	3475	1
7 Stewart Creek Loop	8	9	8	2–3	15	4600	N/A
8 Mt. Jefferson Loop	8	10	7	2–3	19.5	6550	N/A
9 Table Mountain Traverse	8	10	7	2–3	19	2975	32
0 Mt. Moriah	9	10	8	2–3	19	6720	15
3 Charleston Peak: North Loop & South Loop Trails	9	6	9	2	19.5	5750	8.25

te June

4 Summit Trail	9	10	9	3–4	30	7125	12
5 Jarbidge & Emerald Lake Loop	8	8	6	2–4	20	5050	N/A
6 East Fork Jarbidge River & Cougar Creek Loop	8	9	8	4–5	29	5990	N/A
7 Gods Pocket Peak Trail to Camp Creek	9	10	5	2–4	24	5225	N/A
1 Right Fork Lamoille Creek	9	9	7	2–3	9.5	2700	N/A
4 Overland Lake Trail	9	10	9	2–3	12	3300	N/A
1 Baker Creek Loop to Baker & Johnson Lakes	9	8	7	2–3	14	3625	N/A

rly July

1 Tahoe Rim Trail: Daggett Pass to Brockway Summit	8	7	7	4–5	52	8325	36
3 Ophir Creek Trail	7	8	8	2	8	3900	27
8 Winchell Lake Trail	8	9	2	2–3	6	1110	N/A

d-July

2 Mt. Rose & Bronco Creek	8	5	7	2–3	13	3350	N/A
9 Greys Lake Trail	8	7	6	2–3	10.5	3275	N/A
2 Ruby Lakes	10	7	7	2–4	11	2950	N/A
3 Ruby Crest Trail	10	10	7	3–5	34	9700	57

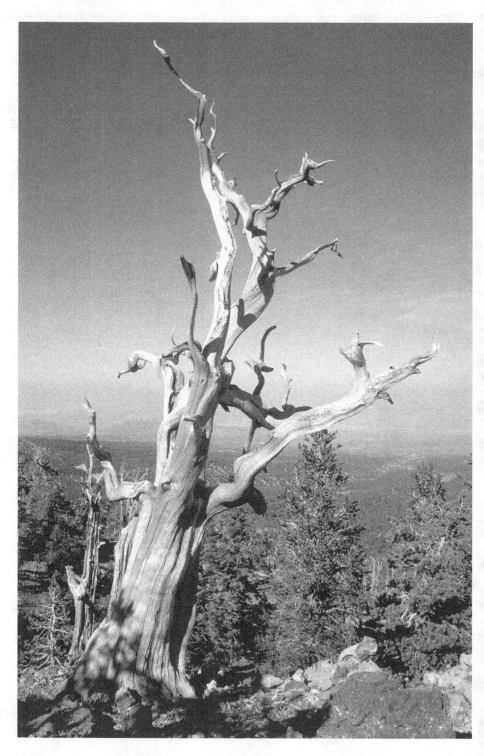

Old bristlecone pine, Spring Mountain (Trip 23)

Introduction

Those unfamiliar with Nevada generally have one of two distinctly different images of the state: a vast, lifeless open space filled from one end to the other with the ubiquitous sagebrush, or a land evoking sensory overload caused by the glittering opulence found on the neon-enriched Las Vegas Strip. The idea of mountains with magnificent wilderness harboring wildflower-laden meadows, clear, rushing streams, alpine lakes, and jagged peaks is beyond the comprehension of most people. Travelers speed across the state on the major highways, the expansive landscape a mere obstacle to reaching their ultimate destination, completely unaware of the extraordinary landscape beyond the asphalt and the bordering sea of sagebrush.

The state of Nevada is the most mountainous state in the Union outside of Alaska, having a basin-and-range topography common to all the Great Basin. Here the typical mountain range is long and narrow with a north-south-trending orientation, bordered on each side by an arid valley. This pattern is repeated numerous times across the breadth of the Great Basin, creating rows of linear mountain ranges, some with summits as high as 13,000 feet that tower thousands of feet above deep basins on each side. Along the spines of these ranges are island sanctuaries harboring diverse ecosystems that differ greatly from those found in the neighboring valleys. Whereas the basins can be extremely hot and inhospitable during the summer, the ranges above, benefiting from additional moisture and cooler temperatures, contain forests, meadows, streams and lakes that attract wildlife and lure recreationists.

While throngs of admiring backpackers compete fiercely over wilderness permits for access into the highly prized backcountry of the Sierra Nevada in neighboring California, most of Nevada's backcountry remains as untrammeled as ever. Due primarily to a remoteness that requires a long drive from the nearest population center, the wild areas of Nevada still provide plenty of solitude and serenity, amid stunning scenery as grand as any in the country. Even within the more popular areas near Las Vegas and Reno, which include the Mt. Charleston and Mt. Rose wilderness areas, visitation

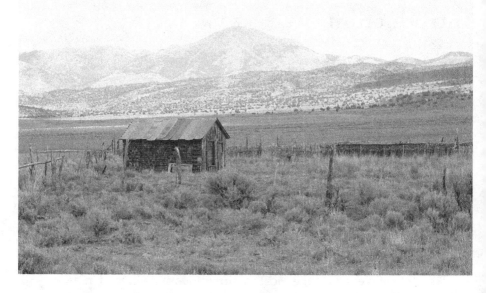

Abandoned cabin in Reese River Valley, Arc Dome in the distance (Trip 15)

is light enough that permits and quotas have never been implemented.

The wild areas of Nevada, where blue skies, clear air, sunshine, and unparalleled vistas abound, have much to offer the adventurer willing to journey away from the more popular areas of the American West. The only scarcity in these mountains is people—no standing in line to beat the quota system for a permit, no competition for the last remaining campsite at a favorite lake, and no crowded shuttle-bus ride through an auto-choked valley to reach a trailhead. For the most part, the landscape remains wild and untamed, a true representative of what wilderness should be.

The 23 backpack trips in this guide represent what the author considers the best backpack trips in the state. Due to the topography of Nevada's mountains, many of these trips are well-suited for a typical weekend or three-day journey, but you will find a number of lengthier trips that could be the basis for a memorable extended vacation. Wherever you decide to visit, may the majesty of Nevada's backcountry fulfill your wildest dreams.

HOW TO USE THIS GUIDE

Each featured trip begins with headings that provide a quick overview of pertinent details to assist you in planning a backpack in Nevada.

Area

This names the specific mountain range or, in the case of Trip 21, the park, in which you'll find the featured trip.

Scenery

This rating is a very subjective evaluation by the author of the overall scenery using a scale of 1 (poor) to 10 (excellent). Bear in mind that such a rating is a relative assessment based on scenic attributes important to the author, and that you may have a different perspective.

Solitude

With a few exceptions, just about any trip in Nevada will provide an excellent opportunity to experience huge doses of solitude. A rating of 10 will generally mean that you have the backcountry to yourself, while a rating of 1 might mean you're sharing your campsite with a horde of boy scouts.

Difficulty

Another very subjective evaluation, this rating assesses the overall difficulty of a particular trip in relation to other backpacks. In general, backpacking is a difficult activity for the average citizen, and even the easiest trip could be considered exceedingly difficult by those unaccustomed to the rigors of carrying all one's necessities on one's back while traveling over mountainous terrain. Most of Nevada's backcountry trails will present some sort of challenge, even to the most physically fit backpacker. A rating of 1 is relatively easy and a rating of 10 is the most difficult.

Mileage

This number is the total mileage of the trip. Mileages in parentheses represent the extra round-trip distance of recommended side trips. Many backpackers may wish to expand the range of their trips even farther, which obviously would mean additional mileage.

Elevation Gain

This figure represents the total accumulated elevation gain over a round-trip course, as opposed to the net gain (elevation gain minus elevation loss). As with the mileage entry, an elevation shown in parentheses is the total elevation gain of recommended side trips.

Days

This figure represents the minimum number of days necessary for the average backpacker to obtain a modicum of enjoyment out of a trip. Incorporated into this evaluation are such considerations as the length of a reasonable day's travel, the spacing of campsites, and the overall difficulty of the terrain. Some parties will undoubtedly want to spend more time enjoying the Nevada backcountry, while super-hikers may blow through a trip much more speedily.

Shuttle Mileage

The approximate road distance between trailheads of a non-loop trip. On certain Nevada backpacks, you will have to do some extra planning to effectively arrange for shuttles.

Map(s)

Every trip will have references for the corresponding USGS 7.5-minute quadrangle maps, which show contours along with geographical features. In some areas, a USFS map may be listed as an additional resource. Each trip has its own map appearing before the description that has been created by the author using the most up-to-date information.

Usually Open

In Nevada, where the timing of winter snowfall can be highly variable from one year to the next, this is a very general prediction as to when a particular trail is apt to be snow free.

Best

The second entry regarding season of use is a general assessment of when the attributes of a trip are at their best. This may be based on the availability of water, the peak of wildflower season or autumn color, or the usual weather patterns.

Permits

This listing is for any permits that may be necessary for entry into the backcountry. At this time, none of the trips described in this book require a wilderness permit.

Contact

This listing is the phone number for the agency that has jurisdiction over the area. You can usually get helpful information on backcountry conditions from rangers with the Forest Service or Park Service.

Special Attractions

This section focuses on the outstanding attributes of a particular area.

Problems

If a trip has any particularly troublesome problems, they will be mentioned in this entry.

Tips

Placed within the individual trip descriptions, tips can help make your trip more enjoyable. They cover various subjects, from possible alternative routes to where you'll find the best views or the nearest water.

Warnings

Also within the descriptions, warnings should help you have a better experience in the Nevada backcountry. They serve as alerts that on a certain trail you may find a dried-up water source, aggressive mountain bikers, an indistinct path, or some other challenge.

Possible Itinerary

At the end of each description is a table listing a recommended number of days for a trip, distances, elevation gains, and the locations of campsites for each day. These recommendations may not be best for your particular party or meet the specific needs of your group. This table should be viewed primarily as a planning tool and not a standard to which any group should rigorously adhere.

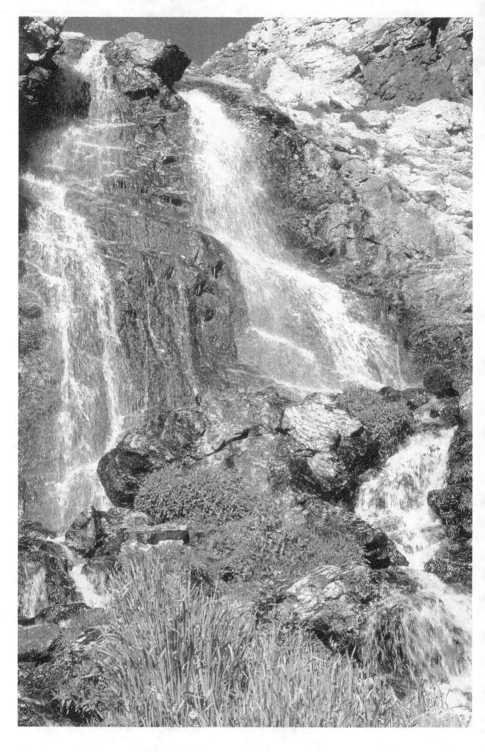

Falls on Overland Creek, Ruby Crest Trail (Trip 13)

General Tips on Backpacking in Nevada

1. Water's being a precious commodity within the borders of the driest state in the nation should surprise no one. The availability of water within the backcountry may vary from year to year depending mostly on the previous winter's snowpack, and will definitely vary from the start of the backpacking season to the end. Always arrive at the trailhead with full containers of water and plan your route carefully. All water acquired in the backcountry should be treated before drinking.

2. Corresponding to being the driest state, Nevada also is one of the sunniest states. Backpackers will need to be prepared for lots of sunshine, oftentimes in combination with high altitudes. Summertime often produces hot temperatures at the lower elevations. Be prepared with plenty of sunblock for exposed areas of skin, sunglasses for the eyes, a hat that provides adequate protection, and clothes that are lightweight, loose-fitting, and light-colored. Avoid more serious problems such as heat stroke, heat exhaustion, dehydration and cramps by maintaining a proper intake of fluids and salts, and by avoiding overexertion.

3. Inadequate funding for trail maintenance and a general lack of use make for very primitive trails within the Nevada backcountry. Away from the most popular routes, be prepared for trails that are overgrown, are in disrepair, or have sections that have disappeared altogether. Many junctions remain inadequately signed, or unsigned. Backpackers planning trips in Nevada should be skilled in navigation, route finding and map reading. Be forewarned that some maps do not accurately portray the actual location of some trails.

4. While a passenger car may be a fine mode of transportation for getting to some of the more popular trails accessible by paved roads, the more remote areas of the state that require long drives on non-paved roads are better negotiated by a more durable vehicle, like a pickup or a 4WD.

5. Trails at low- to mid-elevations in the Nevada backcountry pass through rattlesnake habitat, although the potential for harmful encounters is relatively low. A watchful eye is the best defense against an unexpected meeting between snake and hiker. Actual bites are extremely rare, and serious illness from a rattlesnake bite is even less likely. Stay alert at stream crossings, and along brushy sections near creeks. When venturing off-trail, especially when scrambling over rocky terrain, always watch where you place your hands and feet.

6. Ticks would be considered just nasty blood-sucking pests if not for their potential for causing debilitating disease. In the Nevada backcountry, they are most prevalent in the lower elevations during the spring or early summer, especially after particularly wet winters and springs. In areas where ticks are troublesome, use plenty of repellent, cover up with long-sleeved shirts and long pants with the cuffs tucked into your socks. Self-inspection or examination by a comrade should be done at least once a day. If a tick has burrowed into the skin, use tweezers and apply gentle traction to remove the pest. After complete removal, be sure to wash the area thoroughly.

7. Wilderness permits are not required at this time for backpacking within the national forests of Nevada or within Great Basin National Park. However, especially with the remote nature of much of Nevada's backcountry, where fellow hikers are few and far between and help is generally a long way away, all backpackers should leave a detailed itinerary with a responsible person, complete with instructions about what to do in the event of an emergency.

8. Grazing has been allowed to continue in many backcountry areas of Nevada. Without the mountain ranges to provide summer forage, raising cattle and sheep would be economically unfeasible, according to ranchers whose ancestors have grazed their animals in the same locales for generations. Unfortunately, such grazing has many negative effects on mountain ecosystems. Meadows are trampled, grasslands are overgrazed, and plants are destroyed. Narrow, vibrant creeks become wide, shallow and unhealthy; water quality suffers from the presence of urine and feces. Backpackers in Nevada must be prepared to share the backcountry with cattle and sheep, and the consequences of that presence.

9. The main deer-hunting season in Nevada begins the first weekend in October and continues through the month, preceded by bow and muzzle-loader season. If you travel in the backcountry during hunting season, wear red- or orange-colored clothing.

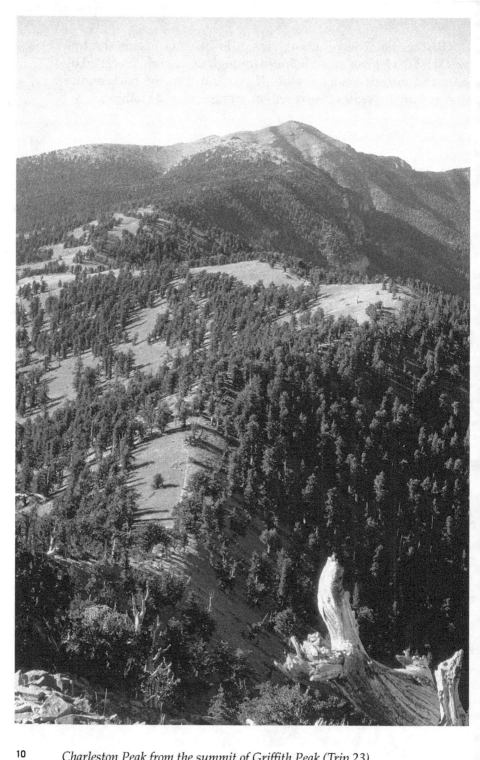

10   *Charleston Peak from the summit of Griffith Peak (Trip 23)*

A Word About Horses

Nevada is perhaps the one place in the American West where those on foot share the backcountry in equal numbers with those on horseback. Away from the more popular trails near Reno and Las Vegas, a chance encounter along the trail with equestrians is as likely as one with backpackers or hikers—that is, not very apt to occur. Along with ordinary equestrians, outfitters regularly use pack animals to escort their paying customers and supplies into the backcountry. The great majority of people you meet in the wilderness will be friendly and considerate, whether on foot or horseback. Unfortunately, just as there is a small percentage of obnoxious backpackers, a similar number of inconsiderate horse users taint the reputation of the rest.

The good news is that since much of the Nevada backcountry receives such light use and the topography is generally well suited for the use of stock, diverse groups of recreationists can compatibly coexist by following a few simple guidelines. To foster cooperation and mutual respect between all users, a list of suggested practices and regulations follows.

Backpackers & Hikers

- Backpackers and hikers should yield the right of way to horses by stepping well off the trail and standing downslope.

Equestrians & Outfitters

- Learn about and implement minimum impact techniques.
- Keep stock to a minimum, using lightweight equipment whenever possible.
- Scatter all manure piles away from trailheads and campsites.
- Choose campsites wisely and tether horses well away from areas of human use.
- Carry pellets or grain (clean feed) wherever overgrazing is possible.
- Keep animals a minimum of 100 yards from any water source.

- Do not tether animals to trees or vegetation for long periods of time—use pickets, nightlines, or hobbles. Use electric fences for temporary corrals and move them regularly.
- Avoid weed-infested areas when riding stock animals or when setting up camp.
- Feed pack animals only weed-free forage for 96 hours prior to entering the backcountry.

In addition to these general guidelines, some jurisdictions have specific regulations governing the use of horses, mules, and llamas. Check with the appropriate agency for current regulations.

Jarbidge Wilderness
- No more than 12 pack or saddle stock per group.
- Use of pellets or weed-free hay is encouraged.

East Humboldt & Ruby Mountain Wildernesses
- Pack in weed-free hay or pellets.
- Use highlines or portable corrals and move frequently.
- Scatter manure.
- No camping with stock at developed campgrounds, or at Greys Lake and Roads End trailheads.
- Groups using more than six horses at one time must pre-plan their trip with the Forest Service.

Great Basin National Park
- Horses or pack animals are prohibited on paved roads, campgrounds, developed areas, self-guided interpretive trails, and day-use zones.
- Horses or pack animals are not allowed within 0.25 mile of the following trails: Bald Mountain Cutoff Trail, Alpine Lakes Loop, Bristlecone/Glacier Trail, Wheeler Peak Trail, Baker to Johnson Lake Cutoff Trail, Osceola Ditch Trail, and Lexington Arch Trail.
- Scatter manure piles at trailheads and backcountry campsites.
- Use weed-free hay for one week prior to visit.
- Do not tie stock to trees or vegetation for any longer than 60 minutes.

- Do not picket, hobble, or allow animals to graze within 100 yards of any lake, stream, or spring.
- Certified noxious weed-free hay is required. Proof of certification for any hay or straw used while visiting the forest or park is required. Visitors using uncertified hay or straw will be fined.

Mt. Charleston Wilderness

- Use pellet feed in the wilderness and prior to arrival.
- The following trails are closed to stock: South Loop Trail, North Loop Trail above Trail Canyon, Bristlecone Trail (except on Scout Canyon Road).

The use of animals in the Nevada backcountry is undergoing review and may be further restricted, to avoid the introduction of non-native plant species. When planning your trip, check with the appropriate agency.

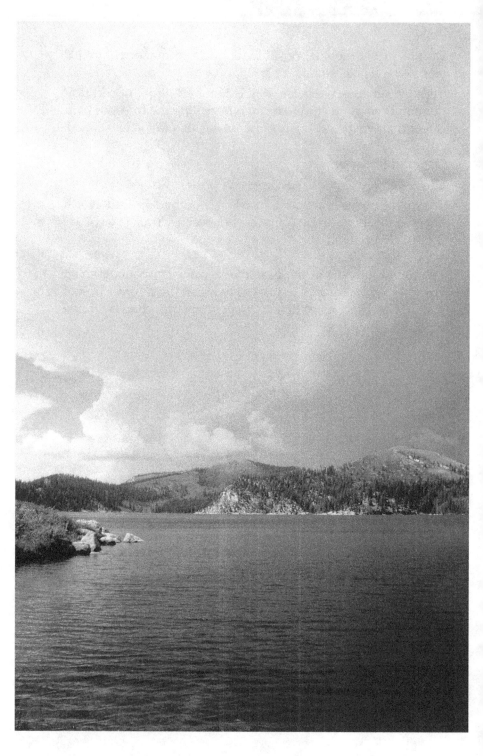

Sky above Marlette Lake (Trip 1)

Wild Areas of Nevada

CARSON RANGE

The Carson Range, a north-south-trending mountain range lying to the east of picturesque Lake Tahoe, is considered a sub-range of the Sierra Nevada. Principally volcanic in geologic composition, the range is a transition zone between the vegetation of the Sierra and the Great Basin, containing plants from both areas. Elevations range from 5000 feet near the eastern base to 10,881 feet at the summit of Freel Peak (inside California), the Tahoe Basin's highest summit. Such a wide elevation spectrum furthers the biological diversity found within the range. Dry, sagebrush-covered slopes, common to much of the Great Basin, are present throughout the area, as expected, but so are lush streamside settings more reminiscent of canyons on the west side of the Sierra. Early summer offers hikers a wide array of wildflowers.

The Carson Range holds the most diverse collection of trees in the entire state. Near the lower elevations is the pinyon-juniper zone, where pinyon pines and western junipers intermix with mountain mahoganies. Next is the Jeffrey-pine-white-fir zone, roughly from 5000 feet to 7500 feet, where you will find smaller amounts of ponderosa pine, sugar pine and incense cedar. Farther upslope, from 7500 feet to 9000 feet, is the red-fir zone, where the namesake tree is found in pure stands or associating with lodgepole, Jeffrey and western white pines, white firs, and mountain hemlocks. Both the red fir and Jeffrey-pine-white-fir zones were heavily logged during the frenzy of the Comstock Lode, in the latter half of the 1800s, and the trees inhabiting the range at present are almost exclusively part of a second-growth forest. The upper forest zone, from 9300 feet to timberline, at 10,300 feet, is the whitebark-pine zone, where groves of whitebarks may contain some lodgepole pine or mountain hemlock. Characteristic of the east side of the Sierra, the Carson Range offers many steep canyons filled with quaking aspen, which become flames of gold in autumn. The Nevada part of the Carson Range boasts a small alpine zone near the summit of Mt. Rose.

The Carson Range is within the jurisdiction of Toiyabe National Forest, and within these lands is Mt. Rose Wilderness, a 28,000-acre parcel toward the north end named after the tallest peak, Mt. Rose, third-highest summit in the Tahoe Basin. The wilderness is split into two pieces divided by the Hunter Lake Road, the 5000-acre Hunter Creek Unit and the 23,000-acre Mt. Rose Unit, which holds the bulk of the maintained trails.

The Carson Range is the backyard playground for residents of Reno-Sparks, Carson City and the Carson Valley towns of Minden and Gardnerville, as well as for visitors and residents of the communities around the east shore of Lake Tahoe. Along with the Spring Mountains near Las Vegas, these mountains experience much more visitation than anyplace else in Nevada; the trail to the summit of Mt. Rose may be the most heavily traveled in the state. Fortunately, this popularity is concentrated in a few areas, leaving much of the Carson Range to be experienced with a reasonable expectation of solitude.

Due to the proximity of an urban center, recreationists will be able to find anything necessary for a backpacking trip into the Carson Range.

SANTA ROSA RANGE

The highlight of the Santa Rosa Range is Santa Rosa-Paradise Peak Wilderness, a 31,000-acre tract of primitive land straddling the range just south of the Oregon border and 35 miles north of Winnemucca. Although one of the smallest designated wilderness areas in Nevada, Santa Rosa-Paradise Peak Wilderness is a treasure. At 9701 feet, Santa Rosa Peak is one of the most dramatic-looking peaks around, especially when viewed from upper Rebel Creek, where you see the peak perched majestically above the aspen-filled basin, a stand of trees that must be one of the largest in the entire Great Basin.

As with most Nevada ranges, the Santa Rosas trend along a north-south axis. Near the crest, rugged granite peaks tower over the surrounding terrain, while the deeply cut, V-shaped canyons along the western base of the mountains reveal a composition principally of phyllite, a metamorphic rock containing small flecks of mica. Ten tumbling, cascading creeks career their way through these winding canyons, from 9000-foot basins near the crest to the

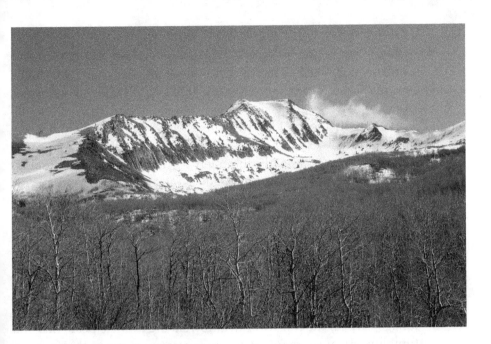

Santa Rosa Peak in spring (Trip 4)

serenely gliding Quinn River in the valley below. Lush, riparian foliage thrives along the banks of these creeks in their lower canyons, while the hillsides above are typically covered with sagebrush and grasses. Farther upstream, where adequate groundwater is present, large stands of aspen fill the canyons.

The east side of the range is considerably steeper, dropping from the crest some 4500 feet to Paradise Valley in 3 short miles. Unlike streams on the west side, the east side creeks plummet rapidly down the precipitous slope toward verdant ranchland in the valley below. Many of the canyons on this side of the range are filled with some of the most luxuriant foliage in the state.

Plenty of wildlife call the Santa Rosas home, including mule deer, mountain lions, bobcats, coyotes, marmots, and a host of other rodents. Reintroduced in the late 1970s, California bighorn sheep have prospered, increasing in number and expanding in range. They may be seen clambering through the rocky terrain in the rugged parts of the upper canyons and along ridgelines. Golden eagles, red-tailed hawks and goshawks are raptors often seen soaring above the canyons in search of individuals from a healthy rodent population. Birdwatchers are apt to spy mountain bluebirds, flickers, wrens and warblers, while sage grouse and chukar are common game birds. The streams provide excellent habitat for rainbow and brook trout, as well as the threatened Lahontan cutthroat trout.

Although a federal highway parallels the range in Quinn River Valley on the west and a state highway in Paradise Valley on the east, the range is a nearly forgotten island of wilderness. Remote and seldom visited, the Santa Rosas are a hiker's haven, with numerous short trails following stream canyons that penetrate the range from east and west. The highlight for backpackers is the 29-mile Summit Trail, a route that crosses the divide at either end to make a lengthy traverse of the east side of the range.

The Summit Trail begins and ends at elevations near 5000 feet, where summer temperatures in the shadeless lower canyons can be quite hot. Early summer may be the best time for a visit, as green foliage carpets the hillsides, wildflowers are at their peak, and the tumbling streams are full. Autumn is also an excellent time to plan a trip, after the hot summer temperatures have moderated and the fall color in the upper canyons of acres and acres of quaking aspen can be quite breathtaking.

A backpack along the Summit Trail is not without drawbacks, as much of the trail is in poor shape, if not missing altogether, particularly the northern section on the east side of the range. Backpacking groups should be skilled in navigation and equipped accordingly. Also, developed campsites are few and far between. A high-clearance vehicle is recommended for the approach to the trailheads.

JARBIDGE MOUNTAINS

As the only wilderness area in Nevada created by the original Wilderness Act of 1964, the Jarbidge Wilderness is an excellent representation of what the authors of the bill had in mind. To the initial 64,830 acres set aside in 1964, the Nevada Wilderness Bill added another 48,500 acres in 1989 for a total of 113,330. Isolated in the northeast corner of the state, far away from anything close to a population center, the tiny burg of Jarbidge is over 100 road miles from Elko, Nevada or Twin Falls, Idaho, the two closest major towns. Adding to the remoteness, many of those miles are over dirt roads. Many more hundreds of miles separate the region from the nearest major cities. Consequently, the Jarbidge Mountains are remote and seldom visited.

A mostly volcanic range, the Jarbidge Mountains seem to share few of the attributes found in the typical Nevada mountain range. While most ranges in the state have a single, north-south trending spine, the mountains of Jarbidge seem to have been dropped from the sky in a clump by the Creator, with many high peaks along multiple crests and deep canyons winding away toward all points on the compass. Eight peaks reach heights over 10,000 feet, and many more approach that altitude, while turbulent streams course down canyons several thousands of feet below. Another rarity in Nevada ranges, two subalpine lakes, Jarbidge and Emerald, nestle near the crests of their respective basins, offering superb destinations for overnight stays.

Positioned just below the Idaho border, the Jarbidge Mountains attract a wealth of winter storms that oftentimes pass to the north of other ranges in the state. These disturbances are usually products of the collision of Pacific cold fronts and warm Gulf air, which produce abundant amounts of precipitation that make Jarbidge one of the wettest mountain ranges in Nevada.

With the additional moisture, extensive stands of subalpine firs and whitebark pines add legitimacy to the Humboldt-Toiyabe National Forest appellation, something of a misnomer in drier ranges within Nevada. Along with these two conifers, other tree species within the area include western juniper, limber pine, mountain mahogany, cottonwood and aspen. Any flower lover will be impressed with the diverse and prolific nature of Jarbidge's wildflowers, as color carpets the hillsides and canyons within the area from June through July. Over forty different species appear between 6500 feet and the upper elevations, creating a wildflower display that is unrivaled in the state.

The Jarbidge Mountains also harbor an abundance of wildlife, so much so that a trip without spotting a number of mule deer seems hard to fathom. A large herd of antelope resides here in summer and fall. Elk, reintroduced a number of years ago, have expanded to over 100 head. According to Forest Service reports, mountain lions and even moose are in the area, but they remain unseen by the majority of hikers. More common are smaller mammals, such as golden-mantled ground squirrels, chipmunks, rabbits, and yellow-bellied marmots. Raptors include golden eagles and red-tailed hawks. Grouse, chukar, and partridge are familiar game birds. Fishing is some of the best in the state for rainbow, brook, Lahontan cutthroat, redband and bull trout.

Due to the long distance recreationists must overcome just to reach the Jarbidge area, the few who make the journey usually spend more time than just a weekend. The trail system is well suited to extended stays, with over 125 miles of trail and many possible connections. Backpackers could easily spend a couple of weeks in the backcountry without retracing their steps or experiencing everything the wilderness has to offer. Unlike many trails within the Nevada system, the trails within Jarbidge have benefited from several decades of protection and are generally well built, well maintained, and appropriately signed at major junctions.

Trails are usually snow free by sometime in June, but fording the rivers and streams at that time may present more of a challenge than negotiating snow-covered trails. Make sure to check with the Forest Service concerning current conditions if planning an early-season adventure that requires fords of major creeks or rivers. By midsummer, daytime temperatures can be quite hot, especially at the lower elevations in the canyons. On a typical July or August day, 90°F-plus is not unusual, so plan on a large dose of sunshine and heat during the height of summer. Despite the passing of the wildflowers, the drying of grasses, and the lowering of stream flows, autumn can be an enjoyable time for a visit, when daytime temperatures are warm, and stands of aspen put on a spectacular show of golden yellow.

The trails of Jarbidge provide many opportunities to witness some of the history from more prosperous days, as many old cabins, mining equipment, and other artifacts that were left behind remain in remarkably good condition. Remember that these objects are cultural resources deserving of your respect and care.

The Jarbidge area remained relatively unknown for quite sometime, which is no surprise considering its remoteness. The only exceptions were a few sheepherders who coveted the rich grasses covering the hillsides for their flocks. In 1908, Humboldt National Forest came into existence and a ranger station was placed in Mahoney, just outside the current town of Jarbidge. That same year, David Bourne discovered gold in the canyon and 1500 miners streamed in, resulting in the boomtown of Jarbidge. In pragmatic fashion, President Taft excluded the town from the National Forest in 1911, thereby allowing miners to have private ownership of the town and surrounding gulches. Even to this day, the town of Jarbidge, along with Bourne, Moore, and Bonanza gulches, remains in private hands as an inholding within Humboldt-Toiyabe National Forest.

An infamous bit of history occurred here in 1916, when the last known stagecoach robbery happened just outside of town. As with most mining communities, eventually the gold ran out in the 1930s, after having produced over 10 million dollars worth in a little over two decades. While the ore disappeared, the town amazingly lived on, although the population never exceeded 200 after the mines closed.

That the town continues to eke out an existence seems somewhat amazing, since just reaching the burg requires a long drive on a narrow, gravel road that careens down a slender canyon some 20 miles from the end of the nearest paved road. Quite a few structures have survived from the bygone days, having been rebuilt after a major fire swept through town in 1919. This "in the middle of nowhere" town offers a couple of saloons, a gas station, a motel, a trading post, and even a bed-and-breakfast. Generally sedate, on weekends during hunting season the town swells to a size reminiscent of the mining boom.

EAST HUMBOLDT MOUNTAINS

Typical of most mountain ranges in Nevada, the East Humboldts trend north-south along a spiny backbone of high peaks for 25 miles southwest of Wells, between Interstate 80 and State Route 229. Hole in the Mountain Peak, at 11,306 feet, is the climax of the range, where Lizzie's Window forms a natural break in the skyline. Second highest is Humboldt Peak, at 11,020 feet, a mere 3.5 air miles away. Much of the remainder of the crest tops out at over 10,000 feet, several thousands of feet above the basins on either side. The rugged nature of these mountains lends a decidedly alpine flavor to the range.

These mountains benefit from the precipitation of Pacific storms that pass over northeastern Nevada but tend to miss the other parts of the state. This favorable weather pattern, combined with the

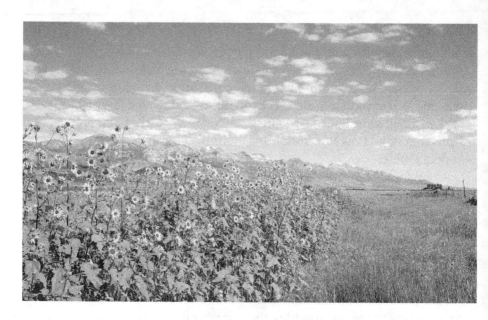

Wildflowers and the East Humboldt Range (Trips 8 and 9)

metamorphic rock in the East Humboldts that tends to hold water near the surface, produces a lush environment that is somewhat unusual for a Nevada mountain range. Backpackers will find abundant wildflowers, verdant meadows, lushly vegetated canyons and healthy stands of limber and whitebark pines.

Plenty of wildlife roam these mountains, but don't expect to see many mule deer, mountain goats, bighorn sheep, or mountain lions from the trail, as these residents are still very timid. More likely, you'll see rodents scampering about, raptors soaring on thermals, or songbirds darting across the sky. The eerie howl of the coyote is often heard around dusk. Fishing for brook, rainbow, and cutthroat trout is good in the lakes and streams.

The East Humboldt Mountain Range is a compact version of the neighboring Ruby Mountains to the southwest, where serrated peaks, glaciated basins, subalpine lakes, rushing streams, and spectacular vistas are all present. Angel Lake, accessible by paved road, is the center of recreational activities here in the East Humboldt Range, where sightseers, anglers, campers, picnickers, equestrians, and hikers all congregate.

Comprising 36,000 acres, East Humboldt Wilderness offers the possibility of an uncrowded backcountry experience away from the relative hubbub around Angel Lake. Whether you desire alpine peaks, cirque basins, deep-blue lakes, wildflower-laden meadows, or aspen-lined creeks, this range won't disappoint. Plenty of opportunities for off-trail exploration will entice cross-country enthusiasts, and mountaineers will find many peaks to bag.

Unfortunately, the East Humboldt Mountains suffer from the same lack of funding for trail maintenance that plagues most of Nevada's backcountry. While the scenery in this range is as spectacular as any in the state, many neglected trails have become overgrown or have disappeared altogether. Paths in the Boulders area, for instance, are so badly overgrown that they should be considered cross-country routes and not bona fide trails, despite their presence on USGS and Forest Service maps.

RUBY MOUNTAINS

Many consider the Rubies the premier mountain range in Nevada. Unlike most Great Basin ranges, the Ruby Mountains exhibit signs of extensive glaciation, including U-shaped canyons, deep cirques holding subalpine lakes, hanging valleys, polished rock walls, and glacier-carved peaks. Of all the mountains within the state, the Rubies are definitely the most alpine-looking, and first-time visitors will most likely be awestruck by such an environment in a state they might otherwise perceive as arid desert. Although the Rubies are some of the best known and most popular mountains in the region, this is still Nevada, where overcrowding is almost unknown. Most of the traffic in the Ruby Mountains, both motorized and human-powered, is concentrated in Lamoille Canyon, leaving the vast, untrammeled backcountry to the hardy few.

The Ruby Mountains were so named in the 1800s, when soldiers from the U.S. Army were sent west to assist pioneers in a search for alternate routes to California. Driven by gold fever, some of the soldiers panned the streams and found garnets, which they mistook for rubies. The name of the gemstone was applied to the surrounding mountains and by the time the error was recognized, the name had stuck. Although incorrectly named, the Ruby Mountains remain the crown jewel of the Great Basin to this day.

The Rubies have two loosely defined regions. The less-visited and smaller section is referred to as the north Rubies, containing the

Soldier Lakes Basin. While there is a smattering of pinnacled summits, this area is characterized by high, open tundra, where one has the sensation of being at the top of the world. A handful of high lakes provides excellent destinations for the relatively few hikers, equestrians, and anglers who venture into the north Rubies.

The central Rubies contain the vast majority of craggy peaks and are blessed with many high lakes and subalpine meadows. Although the central Rubies are made up of a cluster of alpine-looking mountains, much of the range follows a north-south trending ridge between access in Lamoille Canyon to the north and Harrison Pass in the south. The Ruby Crest National Scenic Trail follows this crest for much of that route. The focal point for recreationists and tourists is Lamoille Canyon, accessed by a paved highway.

Lamoille Canyon has been dubbed "the Yosemite of Nevada" and although lacking the spectacular waterfalls and picturesque granite domes of its more famous counterpart, the narrow canyon rewards travelers with exceptional scenic beauty. The scenery includes precipitous slopes rising up to snow-clad and craggy peaks, verdant wildflower-covered meadows, and rushing streams. Several of the area's trails begin at trailheads in this picturesque gorge.

The Ruby Mountains, along with the neighboring East Humboldts, receive more precipitation than most other Nevada ranges. Pacific storms descending from the Pacific Northwest oftentimes miss most of California and Nevada, but brush the northeast corner of Nevada on the way toward the Rockies, transporting additional moisture to the high mountains of the Rubies and East Humboldts along the way. Due to the impervious nature of the metamorphic rock in the area, this extra moisture is held near the surface, replenishing lakes, ponds, streams, marshes, and meadows. Consequently, these two mountain ranges are wetter than most of their Great Basin counterparts.

Predictably, most of this moisture falls as winter snow, but summer thunderstorms are not uncommon, and at times can be frequent and notoriously unpleasant. Quite some time ago, as a newcomer to the Great Basin, the author naively journeyed into the Rubies one summer day sans tent, considering an item of such weight useless in a desert range. Of course, a thunderstorm brewed quickly and poured out its fury, seemingly to scold such arrogance. Fortunately, someone in the hiking party had the foresight to pack a tarp, so everyone got only half soaked.

Lots of wildlife inhabit the Ruby Mountains, although most of the animals are quite wary of human contact. Mountain goats, bighorn sheep, and mule deer are plentiful, while antelope, mountain lions and bobcats are present in smaller numbers. Beavers, marmots, squirrels and other rodents are the mammals most likely to be seen. Raptors like golden eagles and prairie falcons, and game birds, including chukar, partridge, and grouse, are frequently seen in the Rubies. Fishing is excellent for rainbow, brook, and Lahontan cutthroat trout.

TOIYABE MOUNTAINS

The Arc Dome Wilderness at 11,5000 acres is the largest wilderness area in the state, containing the southern third of the Toiyabe Mountains, which are a convoluted grouping of ridges and canyons unlike the mostly linear other Great Basin ranges. Near the north end of the wilderness the mountains narrow to a single spine that continues past the tiny hamlet of Austin. For fifty miles of that length, the crest never dips below 10,000 feet, presenting a massive wall of mountains that rises 4000 feet above the surrounding valleys. Standing majestically over this mountainous domain, the summit of Arc Dome crowns the range, at 11,788 feet, the tenth highest peak in the Silver State.

In the arid center of the state, the lofty Toiyabe Range captures whatever moisture is available from Pacific storms crossing the Great Basin. Consequently, myriad waterways course through the range, including the dubiously named Reese, North Twin, and South Twin rivers. What Mark Twain had to say about Nevada rivers in *Roughing It* seems worthy of repeating here:

> People accustomed to the monster mile-wide Mississippi grow accustomed to associating the term 'river' with a high degree of watery grandeur. Consequently, such people feel rather disappointed when they stand on the shores of the Humboldt or Carson and find that a 'river' in Nevada is a sickly rivulet which is just the counterpart of the Erie Canal in all respects save that the canal is twice as long and four times as deep. One of the pleasantest and most invigorating exercises one can contrive is to run and jump across the Humboldt River till he is overheated, and then drink it dry.

Rainbow over Arc Dome, Toiyabe Range (Trip 15)

The deceptive titles of these watercourses in the Toiyabes were the creation of the Reese River Navigation Company, a scam designed to bilk Easterners out of capital for the development of a steamship system that would transport ore from nearby mines down the "rivers" to processing plants. Despite Mr. Twain's disdain for the term "river" to describe such waterways, the streams within the Toiyabe Mountains are a welcome delight to backpackers, as well as to the native flora and fauna.

The Toiyabes are geologically diverse, as plutonic, volcanic, and sedimentary rocks are all present within the range in significant amounts. Most of the rocks within the Arc Dome Wilderness are volcanic, predominantly of red hues. The steep spines and serrated crests along the rims of the canyons may be leftover pieces of an old crater. Forces of glaciation can be seen around Arc Dome, where deep cirques were carved out of the edges of the broad plateau directly north of the summit.

The large size of the backcountry within Arc Dome Wilderness is a boon for wildlife as well as for recreationists. The range supports a large deer population and, according to the Forest Service, elk have been sighted. Mountain lions, bobcats, coyotes, and beaver also make their homes here, along with the usual conglomeration of

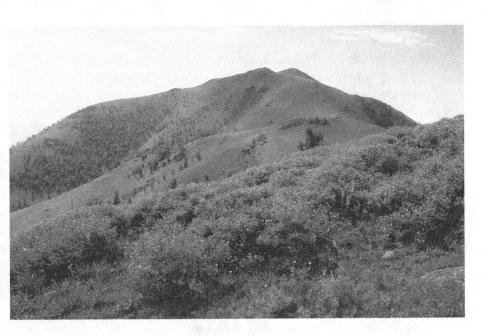

Toiyabe Dome as seen from the Toiyabe Crest Trail (Trip 15)

smaller rodents. Bighorn sheep were once common, but the presence of domestic sheep nearby have limited their range to isolated corners of the wilderness, near the steep crags of South Twin, North Twin, and Jett canyons. Chukar, sage, and blue grouse are common game birds that share the skies with raptors, such as golden eagles, northern goshawks, and prairie falcons. Anglers will find the fishing quite good for native and non-native trout.

In spite of the diversity of wildlife within the Toiyabes, the most often seen animal is the range cow. Even if you avoid the beasts, you probably won't be able to escape the evidence of their presence. Unfortunately, cows oftentimes find appealing the same places that people find attractive, resulting in trampled meadows and polluted streams.

While decent trails are few and far between in many of Nevada's mountain ranges, the Toiyabes have a good network of trails, although more dollars set aside for trail maintenance certainly could improve that network. Truly a backpacker's paradise, several connecting trails allow for the possibility of creating optional trip extensions. A variety of trails lead along stream canyons filled with lush riparian vegetation. However, the highlight of the trail system is the 65-mile-long Toiyabe Crest National Recreation Trail, which offers magnificent vistas and exceptional scenery. The open topography found in the Toiyabes allows hikers with modest cross-country skills to travel off-trail through the range with relative ease.

TOQUIMA RANGE

The Toquima Range, near the geographic center of Nevada, is a linear spine of mountains above two desert basins, Monitor Valley on the east and Big Smoky Valley to the west. As the middle range of three prominent, north-south-trending mountain chains, all with designated wilderness areas, the Toquimas are sandwiched between the Toiyabe and Monitor ranges. In the heart of the Toquima Range is triple-peaked Mt. Jefferson, rising above a unique alpine tableland designated as the 3440-acre Mt. Jefferson Research Natural Area, and site of the highest known Native American village in North America. Soaring above the surrounding valleys, Mt. Jefferson is an imposing figure on central Nevada's skyline, as deep canyons on the north and south separate the crest from the remainder of the range, creating the appearance of a massive bulk isolated above the surrounding landscape.

The 38,000-acre Alta Toquima Wilderness area straddles Mt. Jefferson, affording wilderness protection to the remote backcountry, which beckons the adventurous to partake of the area's unique wonders. High alpine tablelands with wide-ranging views and glacier-carved canyons with tumbling streams are just some of the highlights. Although maps indicate a 50-mile network of trails, many of these paths have become little more than cross-country routes, thanks in part to a lack of funding for trail maintenance and an overall lack of use. An unfortunate maxim of the governance of backcountry trails dictates that trails receiving the highest use also receive the lion's share of funding for maintenance, leaving little-used trails like those in the Toquimas high and dry.

The Pine Creek Trail, the most-used path in this lightly visited wilderness, is a delightful exception. The tread is in excellent condition for the most part, and the route provides a straightforward link to South Summit and the Mt. Jefferson plateau. Once above the canyon, however, the track disappears for stretches, and those wishing to complete the loop as described here will have to be prepared for some off-trail hiking and route finding, although the open terrain is relatively easily negotiated.

The vegetation is typical of central Nevada mountains, with sagebrush and grasses carpeting the lower slopes, pinyon-juniper woodland cloaking the middle elevations, scattered limber pine appearing on the upper slopes, and lush riparian foliage lining the banks of the streams. However, on the plateau a unique variety of desert-alpine flora that includes many endemic species will impress botanists of every level.

The Toquima Range is an interesting area rich in human as well as natural history. The name literally means "black backs," a reference to a band of Mono Indians who once roamed the Reese River Valley. In 1978, archeologists discovered the remains of a village on top of Mt. Jefferson that male hunting parties supposedly used some 7000 years ago. Later, around 1300 A.D., entire families inhabited the site, but scientists are unsure of why they choose to reside here. In more recent times, John Muir explored the area, concluding from his geological evaluation that glaciers played an important part in the formation of mountains within the Great Basin.

Native Americans may have hunted bighorn sheep in the Toquima Range, but early in the 20th century the animals disappeared. Recently, wildlife biologists have reintroduced a small band of desert bighorns, hoping to restore them to their original range. Along with the sheep, the Toquimas are home to deer, mountain lions, coyotes, and a host of small rodents. The plateau offers excellent opportunities to scan the sky in search of raptors, such as golden eagles, northern goshawks, and prairie falcons, riding the thermals above the deep canyons. Pine Creek is the only viable fishing stream, offering the chance to catch rainbow and brook trout.

MONITOR RANGE

The Monitor Range is the easternmost of the three principal central Nevada ranges that lure recreationists. Table Mountain Wilderness straddles the mesa-like high country of the Monitor Range, at 98,000-acres the third largest wilderness area in the state. The Monitors are a classic example of the north-south trending, long and narrow Great Basin mountain range; nearly 115 miles long, they never gain a width greater than about 10 miles.

Although typical in those respects, Table Mountain Wilderness possesses some unique characteristics. At a lofty height, above 10,000 feet, a 12-square-mile tableland is the crowning landmark

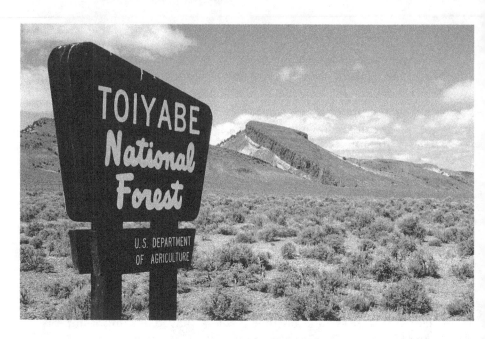

National Forest sign in Monitor Valley (Trip 18)

and namesake of the Wilderness. Covering a significant portion of the tableland are some of the largest stands of quaking aspen in the Great Basin, creating significant swaths of silver-green in summer and blazing gold in autumn. Another distinctive attribute of the area is the large herd of Rocky Mountain elk; transplanted here in 1979. The herd has grown to over 300 individuals.

Besides the elk, the Monitor Range supports one of the largest mule-deer herds in the state. Other large mammals include the mountain lion, bobcat, and coyote. Birds of prey, including golden eagles, northern goshawks, and prairie falcons, patrol the skies above the grasslands and canyons. Important game birds include chukar, blue grouse and sage grouse. Hikers will find plenty of streamside evidence of beaver activity along the five perennial streams that flow away from Table Mountain and out into the surrounding valleys. These healthy creeks provide anglers with excellent opportunities to test their skills on rainbow, brook, brown, and Lahontan cutthroat trout.

While the prolific stands of aspen provide a scenic focal point, other species of deciduous trees and conifers appear in the Monitor Range. Small pockets of limber pine grace the slopes near the crest, typically the only species of pine found in the upper elevations of the mountains between the Sierra and the easternmost ranges of Nevada. In the lower realms, pinyon-juniper woodland, including mountain mahogany and sagebrush, cover the slopes, while cottonwoods tower over the riparian foliage thriving along the stream banks.

The Monitor Range is a remote and seldom-visited region, far from a town of any size. Access to trailheads requires long drives on gravel and dirt roads, many of which may be suitable for passenger cars, although most drivers will feel more comfortable on some of these roads with a high-clearance rig.

The tableland topography and mildly graded trails in Table Mountain Wilderness appeal to both backpackers and equestrians. Over 100 miles of trail form a network covering the plateau and connecting with access trails, providing many possibilities for extended trips and loops of varying duration. Trails are usually snow free and passable by early summer, when meadows are green and wildflowers are blooming. In some ways, autumn is the best time for a visit, when acres of aspen turn gold and the occasional bugle of the male elk can be heard. Whatever season you choose, Table Mountain Wilderness offers exceptional backcountry travel.

SNAKE RANGE

A nearly forgotten northern neighbor of the more renowned Great Basin National Park, Mt. Moriah Wilderness encompasses the north end of the Snake Range near the remote eastern edge of Nevada. Piercing the clear air and deep blue skies, 12,067-foot Mt. Moriah thrusts its summit above the neighboring basins as the fifth highest peak in the state. Immediately northeast of the peak and 1000 feet below, a broad, slightly sloping plateau named The Table is another unique feature of the Wilderness. Bordered by groves of bristlecone pines, sparse, alpine-like vegetation covers the rest of the 7000-acre tableland, allowing expansive views of the surrounding landscape and easy travel across the open slopes.

Composed primarily of quartzite and limestone, metamorphic and sedimentary rocks respectively, the focal point of the northern part of the Snake Range is Mt. Moriah, with its rugged canyons spiraling away from the lofty crest toward Spring Valley to the west and Snake Valley to the east.

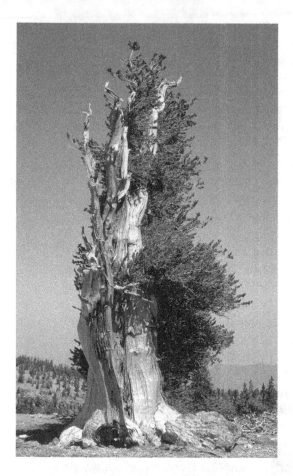

Old bristlecone pine on The Table,
northern Snake Range (Trip 20)

The trails within Mt. Moriah Wilderness pass through some of the most diverse flora in the state, where conifers include pinyon pines, junipers, white firs, Douglas firs, subalpine firs, ponderosa pines, and limber pines, and perhaps the most interesting of all, bristlecone pines. Cottonwoods in the lower canyons and quaking aspen in the higher elevations are well represented also. Autumn color in some of the drainages can be quite dramatic, as in the upper canyon of Hendrys Creek, where quaking aspens fill the basin with golden yellow.

Rocky Mountain bighorn sheep inhabit the steep slopes in the heart of the range. Other mammals include deer, mountain lions, bobcats, coyotes, and rodents. The most frequently seen inhabitants are some of the many species of birds that find their home in the rich and diverse forests. Raptors such as golden eagles, hawks, and falcons can often be seen spiraling up thermals above the deep canyons.

GREAT BASIN NATIONAL PARK

After a long history of struggle, defeat, and compromise, Great Basin National Park became a reality in 1986. Despite the name, this park is more about mountains than basins, harboring subalpine lakes, ice-carved canyons, bristlecone-pine groves, and a bona fide glacier—the only one in the entire Great Basin. Comprising 77,100 acres, the park straddles the crest of the southern Snake Range and includes seven named peaks over 11,500 feet, including Wheeler Peak, second-highest summit in Nevada at 13,063 feet.

One would have to travel all the way across the state to the Carson Range on the east side of the Sierra Nevada to find a range more biologically diverse. Eleven different species of conifer are found in the Snake Range, including white firs, subalpine firs, Englemann spruces, limber pines, pinyon pines, Douglas firs, bristlecone pines and three types of juniper. Great Basin National Park offers three major bristlecone-pine groves, the Wheeler Peak, Mount Washington, and Eagle Peak groves, although the Wheeler Peak Grove is the only one accessible by maintained trail. Some of the most character-rich examples of bristlecones are found within Great Basin NP.

While the Park has several excellent trails leading to interesting destinations, most of them are for dayhikes. Camping is not allowed in the Wheeler Peak and Lexington Arch Day Use Areas, or within bristlecone-pine groves, effectively making the Wheeler Peak Summit, Bristlecone/Glacier, Alpine Lakes Loop and Lexington Arch trails off-limits to overnighters. This leaves trails to Baker and Johnson lakes as the only viable alternatives for backpackers wishing to camp within the Park while hiking on maintained trails. However, the open nature of the topography in the southern Snake Range is well suited for cross-country travel, although the availability of water becomes a significant concern after snowmelt. Mountaineers will find plenty of challenges on the numerous peaks within the Park.

Several other diversions are available to visitors to Great Basin besides back-country travel. A trip to the Park is incomplete without a visit to Lehman Caves, where for a nominal fee you can explore a series of lime-stone caverns on a ranger-led tour. Some of the best campgrounds in the state are also within the Park.

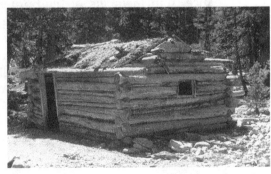

Old cabin along Baker Creek, Great Basin National Park (Trip 21)

SPRING MOUNTAINS

The Spring Mountains are only 30 miles from the Las Vegas Strip, and such natural beauty so close to the glitzy, human-made excess of the casinos presents quite a dichotomy. Aside from the small community of Mt. Charleston, along the Kyle Canyon Road, the Spring Mountains are undisturbed, although if the rapidly expanding tentacles of tract-home development in Las Vegas remain unchecked, houses may soon extend all the way to the base of the range. Currently, a small ski area, hotel, and lodge, along with a grouping of summer homes, are all that interrupt the native surroundings.

Charleston Peak, highest mountain in the range at almost 12,000 feet, was named for Charleston, South Carolina, while the Spring Mountains received their appellation from the many springs bubbling out of the limestone that composes much of the range. Geologists speculate that the formation of the Spring Mountains occurred when limestone deposits, originally under seawater, were thrust-faulted upward several thousands of feet. Nowadays, careful observation can reveal small marine fossils preserved in the limestone.

The 43,000 acres of Mt. Charleston Wilderness are a hiker's paradise, with a wide variety of trails suitable for short to long day hikes. Backpackers will have fewer routes from which to choose, with a definite lack of campsites near water sources. Unlike in much of Nevada's backcountry, the trails within Mt. Charleston Wilderness are in excellent condition, receiving periodic maintenance from members of the Spring Mountain Youth Camp. You won't be spending extra time hunting for trails shown on the map that don't exist on the ground, or trying to fathom the location of an unmarked junction, as might happen in other areas of the state. Mt. Charleston is the most civilized of all of Nevada's wilderness areas.

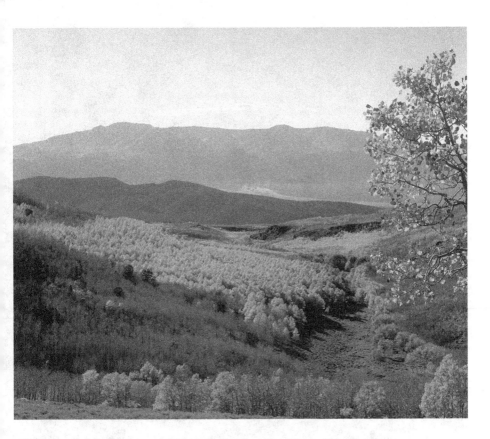

Autumn color from aspen groves on Table Mountain (Trip 19)

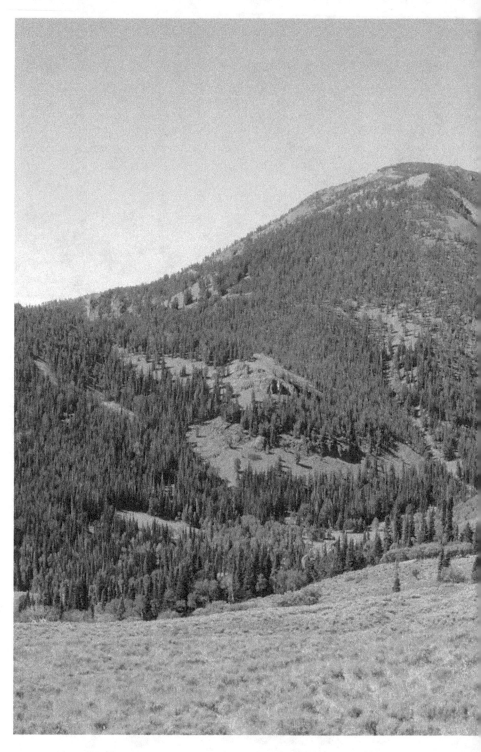

Gods Pocket Peak from the trail, Jarbidge Mountains (Trip 7)

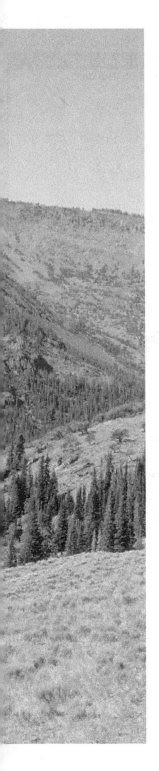

Featured Trips

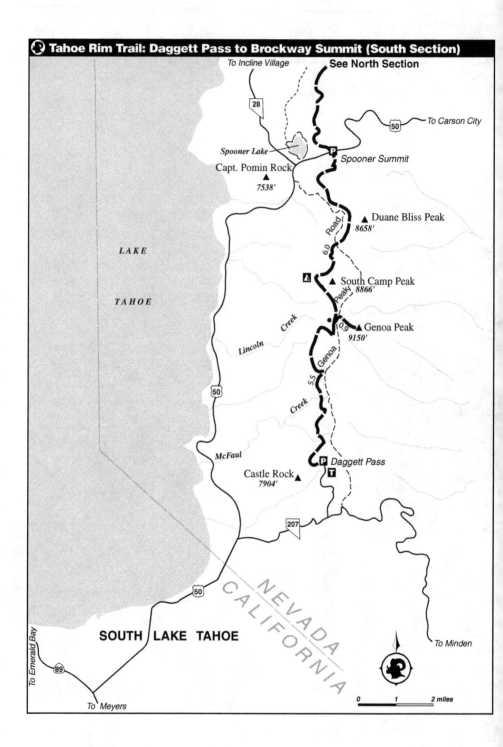

Tahoe Rim Trail: Daggett Pass to Brockway Summit (South Section)

To Incline Village   **See North Section**

28

To Carson City

Spooner Lake   Spooner Summit

Capt. Pomin Rock
▲
7538'

▲ Duane Bliss Peak
8658'

LAKE

▲ South Camp Peak
8866'

TAHOE

Creek

▲ Genoa Peak
9150'

Lincoln

McFaul

Castle Rock ▲
7904'

Daggett Pass

207

NEVADA
CALIFORNIA

SOUTH LAKE TAHOE

To Emerald Bay

To Minden

89

0   1   2 miles

To Meyers

1   Tahoe Rim Trail: Daggett Pass to Brockway Summit

RATINGS (1–10)			MILES	ELEVATION GAIN	DAYS	SHUTTLE MILEAGE
Scenery	Solitude	Difficulty				
8	7	7	52	8325	4–5	36

AREA   Carson Range

MAPS   USGS-*South Lake Tahoe, Glenbrook, Marlette Lake, Mt. Rose, Martis Peak*

USUALLY OPEN   Early July to mid-October

BEST   Mid-July to early August

PERMITS   None

CONTACT   Carson Ranger District (775) 885-6000

SPECIAL ATTRACTIONS   Views, wildflowers

PROBLEMS   Few campsites, lack of water in sections

HOW TO GET THERE   *START (DAGGETT PASS):* Drive on S.R. 207, also known as Kingsbury Grade, to North Benjamin Dr., 0.3 mile west of Daggett Pass and nearly 3 miles east of Highway 50. Turn north and follow North Benjamin Dr. through the homes of Upper Kingsbury. Proceed on the main road, which soon becomes Andria Dr., to the end of the pavement, where you'll find the marked trailhead and a parking area on your left, 1.9 miles from the highway. (No facilities.)

START SECTION 2 (SPOONER SUMMIT): The Tahoe Rim Trail parking lots are on both the north and south sides of U.S. 50, 0.8 miles east

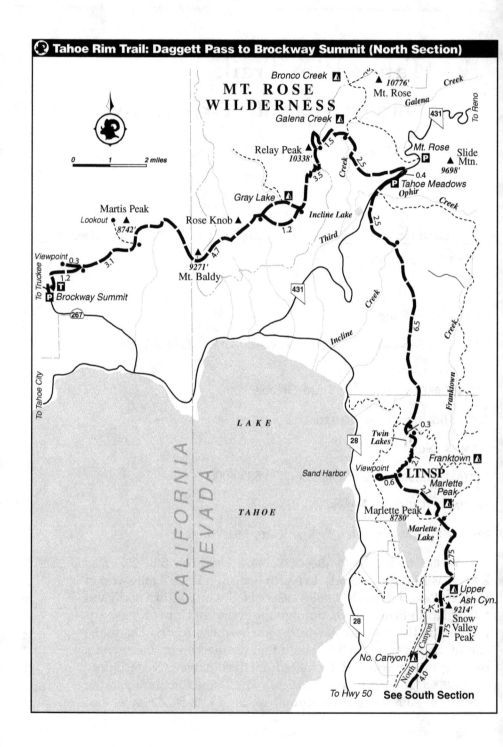

MT. ROSE
WILDERNESS

Bronco Creek

▲ 10776'
Mt. Rose

Creek

Galena

To Reno

Galena Creek

431

Relay Peak ▲
10338'

1.5

Mt. Rose
P

Slide
▲ Mtn.
9698'

2.5

Creek

0.4
P Tahoe Meadows
Ophir

3.5

Gray Lake

Creek

Martis Peak
Lookout ● ▲
8742'

Rose Knob ▲

Incline Lake

1.2

Third

2.5

Viewpoint 0.3
3.1

4.7

9271'
Mt. Baldy

Creek

To Truckee

1.2
T
P Brockway Summit

431

Incline

6.5

Creek

267

To Tahoe City

Franktown

LAKE

Twin
Lakes

0.3

28

2.1

Franktown

Sand Harbor

Viewpoint

LTNSP

Marlette
Peak

0.6

2.7

TAHOE

Marlette Peak ▲
8780'

Marlette
Lake

CALIFORNIA

NEVADA

2.75

Upper
Ash Cyn.
9214'

Snow
Valley
Peak

28

1.75

No. Canyon

North Canyon

4.0

To Hwy 50   See South Section

0   1   2 miles

of Spooner Junction, where 50 intersects S.R. 28. The Spooner Picnic Area on the south side has picnic tables and pit toilets.

START SECTION 2 (TAHOE MEADOWS): At the time of research, the Forest Service had plans for summer 2004 to complete a new trailhead for the Mt. Rose and Tahoe Rim trails near the Mt. Rose Summit on S.R. 431 (also known as the Mt. Rose Highway). Hikers will then have the choice of utilizing the new Mt. Rose trailhead, or the older Tahoe Meadows trailhead. Follow S.R. 431 to the Mt. Rose Summit for the Mt. Rose trailhead, or proceed to the Tahoe Meadows trailhead, 0.7 mile west of Mt. Rose Summit and 7.3 miles east of the junction with S.R. 28, which is in Incline Village. Parking for Tahoe Meadows is available in a lot on the south shoulder, or down a short access road near a building with flush toilets and running water.

END (BROCKWAY SUMMIT): Proceed on California Highway 267 to the TRT parking area, 0.5 mile south of Brockway Summit, and 2.8 miles from the junction with Hwy 28 in Kings Beach. A steep dirt road (FS 16N56) on the west side leads quickly up to a small parking area (no facilities).

INTRODUCTION The completion of the Tahoe Rim Trail has provided hikers, backpackers, equestrians and mountain bikers with a treasure so precious that it's hard to imagine that they've gotten along without the TRT for so long. The section described here, running through Nevada along the east and north edges of Lake Tahoe, offers an abundance of some of the most magnificent views anywhere around the lake. No other section of the TRT stays so close to the crest for so long, allowing numerous bird's-eye views of both the Tahoe basin on one side and the Great Basin on the other. Early to midsummer wildflower displays provide an added bonus. You're apt to encounter a lot fewer people on this section of the TRT as well, especially in comparison to the extremely popular backcountry across the lake.

The Carson Range, being east of the Sierra crest, receives half the amount of annual precipitation that falls on the west side of Lake Tahoe, a mere 15 miles away. Combined with the porous volcanic soils common to the range, the lack of groundwater contributes in part to the sparse forest that allows all those views. Trail users along this stretch of the TRT will face long, dry stretches where water may be hard to obtain, especially as the warm season

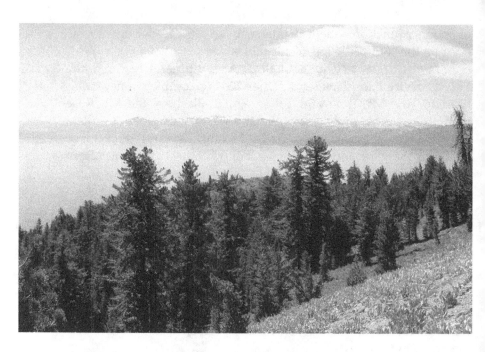

A view of Lake Tahoe from the Tahoe Rim Trail

progresses. Once the annual snowpack has melted, many of the creeks begin to dry up, and some of the few ponds and lakes that do exist on this side of the lake can disappear as well. After snowmelt, the entire first section of this trip, between Daggett Pass and Spooner Summit, may be dry. In the next segment, if Twin Lakes dry up, you may have to travel 17.5 miles from Spooner Summit to trickling Incline Creek before the trail crosses a water source, although with some extra effort, water is available below the crest in side canyons.

An overall lack of water isn't the only concern for backpackers, as decent campsites are also at a premium. In addition, camping within Lake Tahoe Nevada State Park is severely limited to designated campgrounds, which for Tahoe Rim Trail users would be the North Canyon Campground, 1.2 miles west of the TRT, the Marlette Peak Campground, adjacent to the TRT (no water), or the Franktown Creek Campground, 2 miles east of the TRT.

These problems aside, a backpack along the Nevada section of the Tahoe Rim Trail is a worthwhile undertaking. With two major highways traversing the range, shortening the route or completing it in sections are viable alternatives. The incomparable views, vibrant wildflower displays, and high potential for solitude provide the necessary ingredients for a fine adventure.

DESCRIPTION *SECTION 1—DAGGETT PASS TO SPOONER SUMMIT (11.5 miles):* On the TRT, you head up a moderate climb across a shrub-covered hillside, composed of chinquapin, greenleaf and pinemat manzanita, currant and bitterbrush. A sampling of attractive wildflowers adorns the slope in midsummer, beneath an occasional Jeffrey pine or white fir. As the initial climb begins to mellow, you have glimpses of Castle Rock in the foreground, along with a part of Lake Tahoe, and some of the peaks rimming the south shore, including Mt. Tallac and Freel Peak. As you proceed, a thicker forest obscures the view, but quickly you reach a 4x4 post, which marks a lateral leading to a vista point. A short walk along this side path leads to an easy scramble up a rock bluff, from where you won't find the most magnificent lake view along the TRT, but a good look at the south end of Tahoe and the surrounding landscape nonetheless.

Back on the TRT, you proceed through moderate forest cover on a mildly undulating trail, crossing a well-used dirt road at 0.8 mile from the trailhead. For the next several miles, the TRT generally follows the topography, gaining and losing minor amounts of elevation along the way, as the path curves around hillsides and dips into side canyons.

> *Warning:* Early in the season you may find water in seasonal branches of McFaul Creek, otherwise you're in for a long dry haul all the way to the picnic area at Spooner Summit.

Occasionally, the western white pines, red firs and Jeffrey pines of the light-to-moderate forest thin just enough to tempt you with passing glimpses of the lake, providing subtle hints of the incredible vistas ahead.

Nearing the 4.5-mile mark, you curve above the usually dry vale of Lincoln Creek and then drop to the crossing of a well-traveled road in the bottom of the canyon. Reaching the summit of Genoa Peak is possible via this road, but a shorter route is found 0.5 mile farther up the trail. After a moderate, winding 0.5-mile climb, you reach an overgrown old road at 5.25 miles from the Daggett Pass trailhead, which is the start of the shorter route to Genoa Peak.

Beyond the old road, 0.25 mile of gently ascending trail through mixed forest leads to the crossing of a more pronounced jeep road that intersects the Genoa Peak Road after 0.1 mile. Another 0.25 mile of easy climbing away from the road brings you out of the forest to the mile-long crest of South Camp Peak and some of the finest Tahoe vistas to be found anywhere around the lake. On top of a large rock outcrop, a conveniently placed log bench provides splendid accommodations for a lengthy rest stop while you enjoy the view.

Tip: *Tahoe landmarks visible from South Camp Peak are almost too numerous to mention. Make sure you carry a map in your pack that is large enough to cover the entire Tahoe Basin to help you identify the various sights.*

A nearly continuous vista accompanies the easy stroll across the west side of the broad summit, interrupted infrequently by small groves of lodgepole pine and red fir, where campers can arrange for a "room with a view," albeit without water. After the awe-inspiring traverse, another rock outcropping signals the end of the journey across South Camp Peak, beginning the long descent toward Spooner Summit.

A moderate, slightly winding descent from South Camp Peak leads you down a forested ridge, composed initially of lodgepole pines and mountain hemlocks. Farther down, western white pines, red firs and Jeffrey pines replace the conifers of the upper elevations. As you descend, previous logging and slash burning has enabled a healthy population of wildflowers to bloom in early to midsummer. At 8 miles from the Daggett Pass trailhead, you encounter another crossing of Genoa Peak Road, where a sign indi-

Duane Bliss & South Camp Peaks

Ironically, the mountain that currently reveals signs of selective logging on its flanks was named for the co-founder of the Carson and Tahoe Lumber and Fluming Company. Over the course of almost three decades, Bliss and his cohorts devoured most of Tahoe's forest to serve as fuel for the insatiable mining boom of the Comstock Lode. Almost all of the trees now in the Tahoe Basin are part of a second-growth forest, as only a few tiny stands of old-growth forest escaped the denuding. South Camp Peak refers to a logging camp the company established on the west slope of the mountain in 1876.

Much of the recent logging had more noble aspirations. Several years of drought during the early 1990s made some of the conifers susceptible to a bark-beetle infestation. Many of the dead trees were later chopped down and removed in an attempt to promote forest health.

cates that 3 more miles of hiking stand between you and Spooner Summit.

About 0.25 mile after the road, a use-trail angles sharply uphill to a viewpoint on top of a rocky knob, offering a good view down into the Carson Valley. Another 0.5 mile of moderate descent takes you across a jeep road to a milder traverse around the west slope of Duane Bliss Peak. Along the way, the forest offers plenty of reminders of the selective logging that preceded the building of this section of the TRT.

Just beyond the 9-mile mark, you encounter yet another jeep road. A dry campsite nearby offers the possibility of overnight accommodations for those who packed along a sufficient supply of water. The general descent toward Spooner Summit continues through light forest interspersed with pockets of early-season wildflowers, including mule ears, lupine and paintbrush. Sporadic openings in the forest offer lake views along the way, though none as dramatic as those from South Camp Peak. As you begin to hear the roar of traffic along Highway 50, a series of switchbacks herald the descent of the final slope above the Spooner Summit trailhead. A winding descent through sagebrush, tobacco brush, currant and scattered Jeffrey pine and aspen brings you to the paved parking lot of Spooner Picnic Area, 11 miles from the Daggett Pass trailhead.

SECTION 2—SPOONER SUMMIT TO TAHOE MEADOWS (23 miles): From the trailhead, you climb up the hillside away from Highway 50 at a moderate clip through scattered forest that quickly thickens and remains dense for the next several miles. Very infrequent breaks in the trees allow limited views, initially of Spooner Lake and later on of Tahoe, but this section of the TRT is predominantly a shady ascent through thick red-fir and Jeffrey-pine forest. At both 1.3 and 1.9 miles from the trailhead, 4x4 posts mark vista points, where you have rather unspectacular views, made less desirable by the roar of traffic on Highway 50 below. However, at 2.25 miles, another post indicates a more worthwhile scenic diversion via a short scramble over boulders leading to serene views of Tahoe and the mountains above the west shore.

Beyond the vista point, the TRT generally follows the crest of the Carson Range on a more gently graded ascent, through mixed forest cover. At 4 miles, you encounter a signed junction with a trail that drops 700 feet in 1.2 miles to the North Canyon Campground and a junction with the mountain-bike road of the same name that connects Spooner and Marlette lakes.

> **Tip:** *The North Canyon Campground provides TRT backpackers with one of the few alternatives for developed campsites on the east side of Tahoe. Although primitive by most standards, the campground offers a pit toilet, fire pits, sawed logs to sit on, and the opportunity to filter water from the perennial creek nearby. The major drawback is the climb back up to the TRT.*

Away from the junction, a mild climb ensues as open terrain permits views east of Carson Valley and the mountains beyond. Quickly, a switchback directs you back toward the west side of the ridge, where views of the Tahoe Basin offer visual rewards for the previous miles of forested hiking. The beautiful Tahoe vista is briefly interrupted by small groves of trees, but eventually you leave these behind for good to make an angling climb across the open slopes below Snow Valley Peak. Initially the hillside is carpeted with tobacco brush, giving way to sagebrush and bitterbrush on the upper slopes. The views of Lake Tahoe and the surrounding mountains improve with each step.

In a saddle north of Snow Valley Peak, with Marlette Lake below, you reach a junction with a twin-tracked jeep road, designated as Snow Valley Peak Road, 5.75 miles from Spooner Summit.

By descending the left-hand branch, you can reach the North Canyon Road in 1.2 miles, which provides access to scenic Marlette Lake, 0.5 mile up the canyon. Not only is the lake a fine place to swim or filter water, the hillside west of the lake is a botanist's delight, covered with a prolific display of wildflowers in summer and golden aspen trees in autumn. You can avoid backtracking by continuing up the road to the west of Marlette Lake, joining the TRT again at the Hobart Road junction, 0.5 mile southeast of Marlette Peak.

Backpackers who would appreciate a decent campsite with water nearby can follow the Snow Valley Peak Road east into Ash Canyon. A moderate descent from the TRT junction takes you into upper Ash Canyon, where primitive campsites are found along the fringe of the meadows, nestled beneath lodgepole pines.

Tip: A trip to the summit of Snow Valley Peak is a must for every TRT hiker. Simply follow the old road for a short distance and turn right to follow a winding climb to the top, gaining 250 feet in 0.4 mile. The view from atop the 9214-foot mountain is grand, but the topography of the broadly sloping summit requires that you stroll around to take advantage of all the views. Like Genoa Peak, Snow Valley Peak has a microwave tower and equipment, but the vista is well worth ignoring this drawback.

Beyond the junction with the Snow Valley Peak Road, you proceed northbound on the TRT on a short climb over the crest before beginning a mild descent of the ridge directly east of Marlette Lake. Except for a smattering of windblown whitebark pines, the ridge is carpeted with low-growing plants, such as low sagebrush and lupine. Views of Marlette Lake and Lake Tahoe are superb through this section of trail.

The descent becomes moderate where a series of switchbacks begin, and an increasing number of western white pines and red firs start to inhibit the view. At 1.9 miles from the Snow Valley Peak Road junction, you briefly break out into the open again, where the TRT follows a jeep road for 100 yards or so, before angling away and heading back into the trees.

Tip: If water is of critical concern, you can head southwest on this road down a gully. After 0.25 mile, where the road bends northwest, leave the road and continue down the gully for approximately 200 yards to a spring-fed rivulet.

Marlette Lake is Born

Marlette Lake was created in the summer of 1872 when D.L. Bliss and H.M. Yerington, co-owners of the Carson and Tahoe Lumber and Fluming Co., constructed a dirt-fill-and-stone dam across Marlette Creek. The lake was later named for Seneca Hunt Marlette, a New York native who obtained a civil-engineering degree, migrated west and eventually served as the surveyor general for both California and Nevada. From the dam, water from Marlette Lake was diverted into a flume, which traveled 4.75 miles north to enter a 4500-foot tunnel, carved out of the bedrock below the crest of the Carson Range and descending southeast. From there, the water dropped into a second flume, sinuously traveling to a terminus on a ridge near Lakeview. Here the water entered a pipe, and after a nearly 2-mile descent, was propelled 5 miles uphill to another flume, which delivered Gold Hill's and Virginia City's water supply to a reservoir near the crest of the Virginia Range.

The design and construction of this water system was quite an engineering feat at the time, a testament not only to the engineers and builders, but to the incredible bonanza generated by the Comstock Lode. Although the mines were played out long ago, a more recent bonanza has swept the area. With the aid of volunteers, the Flume Trail was cleaned up and repaired, and nowadays is considered one of the premier mountain-bike trails in the nation, offering stupendous views of Lake Tahoe and a very pleasant grade of 40 feet per mile.

After a brief climb, you follow a winding descent to a well-marked junction with the Hobart Road, 2.75 miles from the junction with Snow Valley Peak Road.

Warning: From this point to Tunnel Creek Road, you may encounter mountain bikes along the TRT.

Continue north on the TRT for 0.3 mile to the south junction with the semi-loop trail that arcs around the west and south sides of Marlette Peak. The quandary at this point becomes which way to proceed. If a campsite is your immediate concern, continue on the right-hand branch 0.2 mile to the Marlette Peak Campground, where you'll find a pit toilet and picnic tables, but no water and none within easy reach. Although the left-hand branch is ultimately 0.25 mile longer, you'll experience more scenic views in that

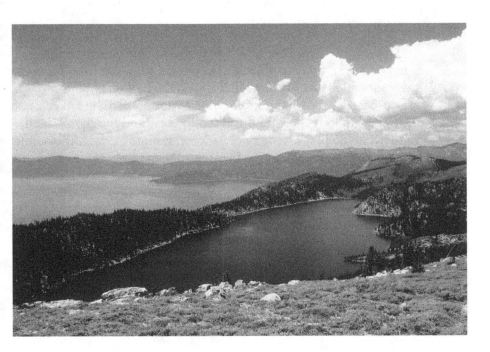

Marlette Lake and Lake Tahoe as seen from the Tahoe Rim Trail

direction via a path closed to mountain bikes. Whichever way you decide to go, the trails reunite north of Marlette Peak, 1.2 miles from Marlette Peak Camp.

From the north junction, the TRT climbs north and then west to gain the Carson Range crest on an open ridge, where a path heads quickly south to another viewpoint providing an excellent vista of Marlette Lake and Lake Tahoe, as well as Marlette and Snow Valley peaks.

Continue west to skirt a rocky knoll and then head north on a forested traverse to a junction with Christopher's Loop Trail, about 1 mile from the previous vista point.

> **Tip:** *Many hikers proclaim the view from the overlook on the west slope of Herlan Peak the best view of Lake Tahoe accessible by trail. The round trip is 1.2 miles and well worth the effort. After the initial switchbacking ascent, the grade eases and the views begin, climaxing at the edge of a granite cliff, where you gaze straight down nearly 2500 feet to Sand Harbor below.*

From the junction, you make a short climb around the south and east sides of Peak 8766 before a steady, zigzagging descent propels you on toward Twin Lakes. Although most of the descent is through a mixed forest, you are afforded occasional views of Lake Tahoe to the west and ahead toward Mt. Rose. At the bottom of your moderate descent, you reach the shore of the easternmost Twin Lake. Light groupings of lodgepole pine and red fir surround the shore, but the sandy soil displays a distinct lack of ground cover. Above the lakeshore, clumps of tobacco brush and manzanita spread beneath the conifers. Since the lakes are within the state park boundary, camping is not allowed.

Warning: *Set in a shallow basin rimmed by ridges and hills, Twin Lakes have no natural inlet or outlet, being dependent upon snowmelt for their existence. Following dry winters, the lakes typically disappear by midsummer — don't plan on finding water here after July.*

Continuing on the TRT, you head away from the lake through a mixed forest of western white pines, lodgepole pines and red firs, quickly encountering a crossing of the well-marked Tunnel Creek Road.

Warning: *Mountain bikers heavily use this road as a connector between the popular Flume Trail and other roads and trails within the state park, including the TRT. North of Tunnel Creek Road, mountain bikers are supposed to have access to the TRT only on even days of the month.*

Tip: *By traveling 2 miles east on the Tunnel Creek Road, you can reach legal camping within the state park at the primitive Franktown Creek Campground, 1100 feet below the TRT. Water is available from the creek nearby.*

Away from the busy road, you make a brief ascent, followed by a lengthy traverse across the west slope of Peak 8437. Through the cover of a fir forest, you unceremoniously exit the state park and proceed through the lands of Toiyabe National Forest. About 2 miles from Tunnel Creek Road, you regain the crest of the Carson Range at a saddle above the canyon of Tunnel Creek, 0.3 mile southeast of Peak 8703. Thirsty backpackers can descend the Tunnel Creek drainage for about 0.25 mile to secure water.

A moderate switchbacking climb leads you out of the saddle and up to a spectacular eastern view, which includes the narrow ribbon of Little Valley below, Washoe Lake nestled into the floor of Washoe Valley in the middle distance, and the desert hills of the Virginia Range beyond. After a half-mile traverse along the east side of the ridge, you cross over to the west side, a pattern that becomes rather frequent over the course of the next several miles. Another 0.25-mile traverse, this time on the west side of the crest, brings you into a minor saddle around 8300', with fine views to both the west and the east. A 0.25-mile stretch along the west side of the ridge brings you to yet another saddle along the crest, at the terminus of a chairlift near the boundary of the Diamond Peak Ski Area.

For the next few miles, the TRT closely follows the crest of the ridge, sometimes on the east side and sometimes on the west side, traversing from one minor saddle to the next. The scattered-to-light forest allows exceptional views alternating between the lovely Tahoe Basin to the west and the dramatic desert lands to the east. The fine views, combined with the mildly graded, slightly rising trail, create an extremely pleasant hiking experience that is so rewarding that you can't help but wonder why this stretch of the TRT is of such recent origin.

Continuing on a northbound course, the TRT slips away from the crest a bit to traverse the canyon holding the headwaters of Incline Creek. Excellent Lake views continue as you follow the trail around the head of the basin. At least one branch of Incline Creek is a fairly reliable source of water in all but the driest of years. Even then, a short jaunt downstream should lead you to water in this spring-fed creek. Early summer will provide a bonus of vibrantly colored wildflowers amid the willows and aspens that line the banks.

From the crossing of Incline Creek, the Tahoe Meadows trailhead is another 2.5 miles. Lake Tahoe remains the centerpiece of the scenery for a while longer, at least until you enter a thick forest of lodgepole pines, as you begin a steeper descent toward Tahoe Meadows. Nearing the meadows, the grade eases and you encounter a well-signed junction with the Ophir Creek Trail, 1 mile from the trailhead. You come to another junction, 0.3 mile farther, between the continuation of the old roadbed heading toward the highway and the newly built section of the TRT angling north toward the trailhead.

Remaining on the TRT, you quickly break out of the trees, hop across gurgling Ophir Creek, and then begin a mild ascent across the green expanse of verdant Tahoe Meadows. Backdropped nicely by 9698-foot Slide Mountain, you'll find that Tahoe Meadows is one of the most scenic subalpine meadows in the northern Sierra, despite the presence of a state highway near the fringe. Early-season hikers will enjoy a wide range of wildflowers, although the ground can be quite boggy then. Species you can expect to enjoy include buttercup, shooting star, penstemon, elephant head, marsh marigold, paintbrush and large-leaved aven. After the long, dry haul along the Carson Range crest, this lush meadowland produces sensory overload. All too soon, you draw near the Mt. Rose Highway and stride just below the busy thoroughfare for the last 0.5 mile to the Tahoe Meadows trailhead.

SECTION 3—TAHOE MEADOWS TO BROCKWAY SUMMIT (18 miles): Unless a new connector trail is built, you must walk 0.4 mile up the Mt. Rose Highway from the Tahoe Meadows trailhead to the resumption of the TRT on the opposite shoulder, where the route follows a service road accessing the microwave equipment on top of Relay Ridge.

From the highway, pass around the closed access gate and start hiking along the sandy road, quickly encountering a wilderness signboard and trail register.

> **Warning:** Since you're still miles from the Mt. Rose Wilderness boundary, mountain bikes are permitted on the road—keep a watchful eye for mountain bikers zooming down from the trailhead to the top of Relay Ridge.

As you climb along the well-graded road, stands of lodgepole pine alternately block and allow increasingly fine views to the southwest of Tahoe, adorned by the distant peaks of Desolation Wilderness. Below is the verdant swath of Tahoe Meadows, where Ophir Creek, glides serenely along before beginning a raucous tumble down the canyon to the east, toward an eventual union with Washoe Lake in a basin below the Virginia Range. As you continue up the road, privately owned Incline Lake bursts into view, just west of the highway. Where your road arcs to the north around Tamarack Peak, you enter deeper forest cover, leaving the views behind. Continue the ascent along the road, passing a small pond near the head of Third Creek on the left and then the junction with the trail to the summit of Mt. Rose on the right, 2.5 miles from the highway.

> **Tip:** Campsites can be found less than 0.5 mile down the Mt. Rose Trail, near the headwaters of Galena Creek.

Just past the Mt. Rose trail junction, the road crosses piped, spring-fed Third Creek and you begin a steeper ascent of the slope below Relay Ridge. Near the base of the tramway tower that services the facilities on the ridge, you follow the road around a sharp bend, and after 0.5 mile double back sharply to switchback up the hillside. As you gain the crest near a plethora of electronic equipment, 4 miles from the highway, Boca, Stampede and Prosser reservoirs spring into view, as does the town of Truckee, backdropped nicely by Donner Lake, as well as the mountainous terrain around Donner Summit.

Entering the Mt. Rose Wilderness, you now follow single-track trail south-southwest along Relay Ridge on a stiff, 0.25-mile climb past wind-sculpted whitebark pines to the top of Relay Peak, where a cairn and an old wooden tripod mark the summit. At 10,338 feet, Relay Peak is the highest point on the entire circuit of the TRT. The stunning vista includes a good portion of Lake Tahoe basin, Tahoe Meadows and Incline Lake below, a piece of Washoe Lake through the gash of Ophir Creek canyon, with a parade of distant ranges extending east into the Great Basin. The Sierra Buttes dominate the northern skyline, but on clear days you should be able to make out Lassen Peak beyond, and on the clearest of days, Mt. Shasta. Unfortunately, the view is not all good, as immediately to the northwest you'll see the results of the extensive Martis Fire of 2001, sparked by an illegal campfire at the hands of careless campers.

Away from Relay Peak, you head down the crest of the ridge for 0.5 mile, before a series of switchbacks leads down the southern flanks of the peak on a protracted descent toward a significant saddle, losing 800 vertical feet in the process. Along the way, you have excellent views of the Donner Summit region, the seldom-traveled terrain of the West Fork Gray Creek, and in the northwest the trio of reservoirs on the Truckee River system and the distant plain of Sierra Valley.

More switchbacks lead to easier hiking as you approach the rocky flanks of Slab Cliffs. Nestled in the small basin below you, at the head of a branch of Third Creek, is Ginny Lake, a pleasant-looking body of water only 0.25 mile from the trail, but virtually inaccessible without a steep, off-trail descent. Continuing, you pass through scattered conifers as you traverse across the rock outcroppings of Slab Cliffs, with more fine views as your nearly constant

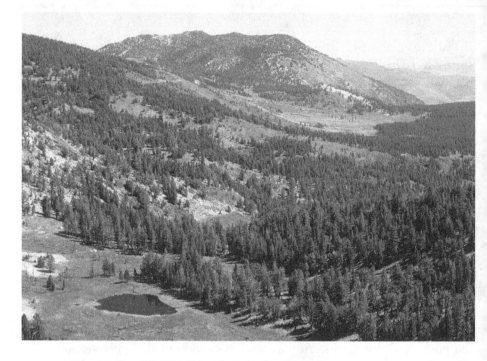

Ginny Lake with Slide Mountain in the distance

companion. Away from Slab Cliffs, a lone switchback drops you into the next saddle along the ridge crest.

A series of short switchbacks leads you down from the saddle to an unmarked junction with an unmaintained section of the old Western States Trail, where faint tread heads east to the private property around Incline Lake. Just downslope, a spring near a pocket of willows provides a reliable water source for most of the summer. Remaining on the TRT, you traverse the open hillside with exquisite views of Lake Tahoe, and in 0.25 mile come directly above aptly named Mud Lake. Without a natural inlet or outlet, the brown pond of Mud Lake stagnates in its basin, progressively shrinking over the course of the summer, and in some years disappearing altogether. Another 0.25 mile of gently graded trail brings you to yet another saddle along the crest, where nearby you'll find a junction with the old Western States Trail to Gray Lake, 7.5 miles from the Mt. Rose Highway.

Side Trip to Gray Lake: Unless you're in a hurry, the half-mile descent to Gray Lake is worthwhile, especially if you need a campsite. Leave the TRT and descend away from the ridge on a section of the old Western States Trail, initially through whitebark pines and mountain hemlocks. In the midst of the descent you cross a small, flower-filled meadow and then continue to drop through a thicker forest of lodgepole pine. After hopping across the thin ribbon of a seasonal stream, you reach the floor of the small basin and meadow-rimmed Gray Lake.

Gray Lake is a kidney-bean-shaped, shallow body of water surrounded by verdant meadows. The lake is destined eventually to become a part of Gray Meadow, as only time is necessary for silt and debris to fill the basin. On a human timetable, however, many years are left to enjoy this delightful lake. The sparkling, spring-fed water of the inlet flows down from above the lake along a rocky channel softened by rich, green moss and brilliant wildflowers. At the head of the canyon the gray, volcanic rock of Rose Knob Peak forms a stark, background for the vibrant meadows. Over the years, numerous avalanches have swept down the side of Rose Knob Peak, delivering an ample supply of timber to the slopes at the base of the peak.

The area around Gray Lake is devoid of any established campsites due to lack of use, although an increase in campers is sure to follow the recent completion of the TRT. Firewood seems plentiful. Swimming looks less than desirable, but anglers may find the fishing good. Further exploration of Mt. Rose Wilderness is possible via the obscure trail that follows the West Fork Gray Creek, although you will ultimately encounter burned areas from the Martis Fire.

To return to the TRT, you have the option of retracing your steps or ascending the moderately graded trail southwest from the lake to a connection with the TRT west of Rose Knob Peak, 1.2 miles from the first junction. **End of Side Trip**

From the first junction to Gray Lake, the TRT skirts the east side of Rose Knob Peak, where excellent lake views abound. You continue to traverse around the south side of the peak through scattered hemlocks and across talus-covered slopes before dropping to a saddle directly west of the peak, where a sprinkling of whitebark pines greets you.

Heading away from the saddle, you traverse the ridge crest over to the junction with the western branch of the old Western States Trail to Gray Lake, 8.9 miles from the highway. The long traverse continues across mostly open slopes, where proclaiming the excellent views becomes redundant. Lake Tahoe glistens under the typically sunny Sierra skies, while Incline Village, the Diamond Peak Ski Area, and the Mt. Rose Highway all lie at your feet. You skirt the slopes below Rose Knob—if even grander views are desired, you can make the 300-foot climb to the top—and continue the traverse across hillsides carpeted with mule ears through midsummer. Passing below unnamed Peak 9499 and 9271-foot Mt. Baldy, you reach the Mt. Rose Wilderness boundary amid scattered pines and then make a mild descent to an unceremonious crossing of the Nevada-California border.

A short zigzagging descent follows the long, open traverse leading you down to a rock knob, from where you have another good lake view. A few switchbacks drop you past some rock cliffs to a 0.75-mile descending traverse of a northwest-trending ridge, from where you are allowed occasional vistas of the lake and the impressive mountainous terrain of the North Tahoe area. A scattered, mixed forest along the ridge begins to thicken toward the end of the traverse, where the trail leaves the ridge to make a moderate descent to a saddle.

From the saddle, a half-mile of easy trail through open areas of rock alternating with stands of forest brings you to a jeep road. The TRT follows the course of this road for about 0.4 mile before single-track trail resumes.

> **Tip:** *Hikers interested in gaining the bird's-eye view from the lookout on Martis Peak can continue on the jeep road for 0.2 mile to a junction with the paved Martis Peak Road (F.S.16N92B). Turn right and head uphill, following the paved road for 0.7 mile to the lookout, perched on a small flat, 0.1 mile northwest of the true summit. Along with the restored lookout, you'll find a picnic table and an outhouse. Thanks to the paved road, you may also find tourists as well. At one time, Martis Peak was the only staffed fire lookout in the Tahoe Basin.*

Leave the jeep road and descend on the single-track trail, quickly leaving the forest to break out into a sloping meadow carpeted with mule ears. A short way beyond the meadow, you curve around the south ridge of Martis Peak and encounter a rocky viewpoint. Once again, the TRT hiker is blessed with a supreme vista of the Lake Tahoe basin. You see not only almost the entire lake, but the major summits surrounding the lake as well.

Tearing yourself away from the beautiful view, you descend moderately back into scattered-to-light red-fir forest, interrupted by another clearing filled with mule ears and farther on by a patch of head-high tobacco brush. At 2.25 miles from the Brockway Summit trailhead, you hop over a thin ribbon of water trickling down the hillside, where wildflowers, grasses and clumps of willow add a splash of vegetation that contrasts vividly with the otherwise dry surroundings. Beyond the thin rivulet, milder trail takes you through selectively logged forest, followed by a more moderate descent that leads to the crossing of well-graded gravel F.S. Road 16N33, just 150 yards southeast of the junction with paved Martis Peak Road.

After crossing the road, just over a half-mile of easy hiking brings you to a junction with a spur trail to the top of Peak 7755. A mildly graded 0.3-mile ascent takes you through trees and shrubs, including chinquapin, tobacco brush and huckleberry oak, up to a pile of rocks at the top of a hill. After the spectacular vistas previously encountered, this view seems fairly pedestrian. However, one last look at the lake may be warranted before you descend the last viewless mile of trail to the trailhead.

From the junction, 1.2 miles of hiking remain, as you follow the TRT on a moderate descent through a selectively logged forest of mainly white firs, with a few Jeffrey pines. As you near the Brockway Summit trailhead, a trio of switchbacks leads you down the hillside above California 267, past the TRT signboard, and out F.S. Road 56 to the highway.

POSSIBLE ITINERARY

	Camp	Miles	Elevation Gain
Day 1	South Camp Peak (dry)	7.0	1000
Day 2	Upper Ash Canyon	9.25	1950
Day 3	Incline Creek	14.5	2775
Day 4	Gray Lake	11.0	2050
Day 5	Out	9.6	550

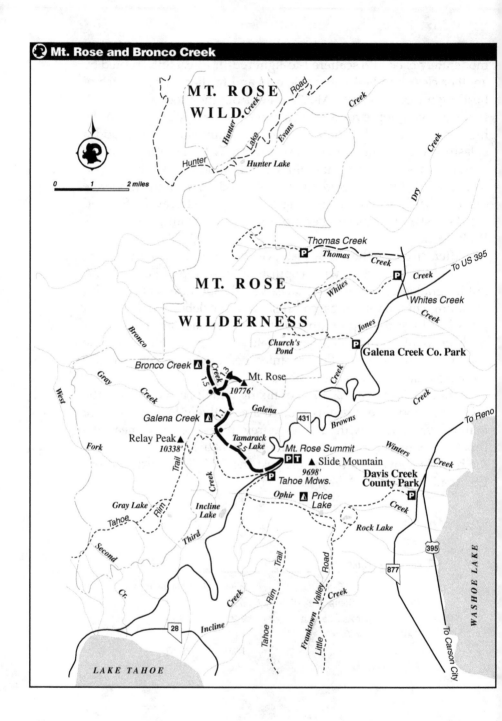

2 Mt. Rose and Bronco Creek

RATINGS (1–10)			MILES	ELEVATION GAIN	DAYS	SHUTTLE MILEAGE
Scenery	Solitude	Difficulty				
8	5	7	13	3350	2–3	N/A

AREA Carson Range

MAPS USGS-*Mt. Rose*

USUALLY OPEN July to mid-October

BEST Mid-July to early August

PERMITS None

CONTACT Carson Ranger District (775) 885-6000

SPECIAL ATTRACTIONS Views, wildflowers

PROBLEMS Poor campsites

HOW TO GET THERE From Reno, take U.S. 395 to the Mt. Rose Highway (State Route 431) and travel west to the Mt. Rose Summit (8911 feet) and the new trailhead which, at the time of research, the Forest Service was hoping to complete in 2004. From Incline Village, the parking area is 8 miles east of the 28/431 junction. The old Mt. Rose trailhead is 0.3 mile west of the summit, where the route of the Tahoe Rim Trail now follows the access road to Relay Ridge.

INTRODUCTION The route to the summit of Mt. Rose may be the most popular trail in the state of Nevada. If not, it certainly ranks near the top of the list. The newly constructed parking lot may be full on weekends. A string of cars used to line the shoulder of the Mt. Rose Highway near the old trailhead during the summer, with a corresponding string of hikers spread out along the trail. The attractions are many, including some spectacular views of Lake Tahoe from the

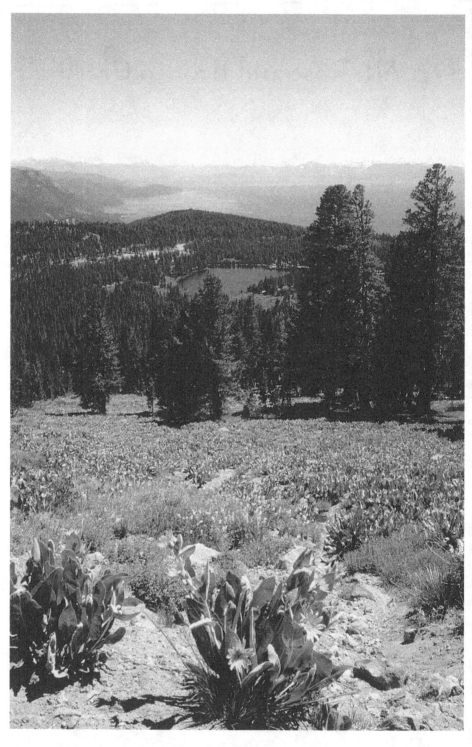

Mule ears, Incline Lake, and Tahoe from the Mt. Rose Trail

summit, a delightful display of wildflowers in the Galena Creek drainage, and the chance to scale the third-highest peak in the Tahoe Basin.

The path to Bronco Creek beyond the Mt. Rose junction is the antithesis of the summit route. If hundreds travel up the trail to Mt. Rose on a summer weekend, you may have to wait a decade or more to see that many people on the Bronco Creek Trail. Rather than excellent views *from* the summit, this trail offers a fine view *of* the summit, from 2000 feet below. A base camp along Bronco Creek allows lonesome exploration of this little-used corner of the Mt. Rose Wilderness. Whether you're searching for alpine heights or meadow lowlands, this trip has plenty to offer.

DESCRIPTION From the parking lot at Mt. Rose Summit, follow new trail on an ascending traverse above the Mt. Rose Highway across a sagebrush- and grass-covered hillside dotted with boulders and sprinkled with lodgepole and whitebark pines. Mule ears and lupines add dashes of purple and yellow to the slopes in early to midsummer. As you continue the climb, the pines become even more widely scattered, which allows for fine views of the upper end of Tahoe Meadows and of Lake Tahoe, rimmed on the far shore by towering peaks. Eventually the trail veers away from the highway and enters light forest on the way to a saddle between Tamarack Peak on your left and Peak 9201 on your right.

Beyond the saddle the gently rising trail slices across the eastern flank of Tamarack Peak, where mountain hemlocks begin to intermix with the pines. Gaps in the trees permit periodic glimpses of meadow-rimmed Tamarack Lake 400 feet below, and the reddish-gray, volcanic summit of Mt. Rose looms above the treetops.

Near the 1.5-mile mark the climbing ends and you begin a mild descent across steep slopes on the northeast side of Tamarack Peak. After the crossing of a seasonal creek, proceed across a forested bench before continuing the descent across another steep hillside. Soon the pleasant sound of running water propels you onward toward a waterfall. Reach the floor of Galena Creek canyon at 2.3 miles from the trailhead and stand below this scenic gem, where multiple ribbons of water spill picturesquely down dark rock walls. Downstream, an expansive meadow provides a fine foreground view for the massive hulk of Mt. Rose.

The Salvation of Galena Creek

Many years ago, the tranquility of Galena Creek canyon was in jeopardy of being lost to the development of a destination resort. Builders would have replaced the beautiful meadows surrounded by stately lodgepole pines with condominiums, golf courses, a ski area and even a casino. Thankfully, a land exchange was worked out between the government and developers, leaving the area in a pristine state.

Away from the fall you cross the creek and skirt the base of a rock-strewn hill opposite the willow- and flower-lined creek and lush meadow to the right. A moderate climb leads away from the creek and meadow and winds uphill to the crossing of a small tributary stream. A short walk from the stream brings you to a junction with the old section of the Mt. Rose Trail, 2.5 miles from the trailhead.

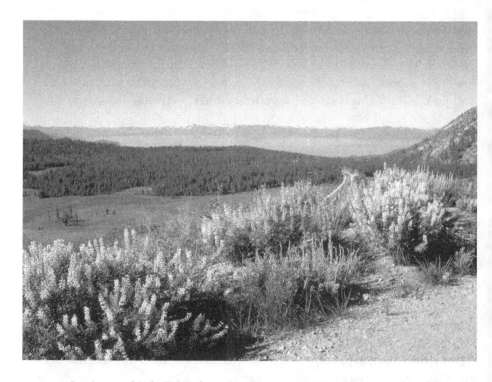

Lupines and Lake Tahoe from the Mt. Rose Trail

From the junction, curve around and cross another tributary of Galena Creek, where an uninterrupted climb to the summit begins. During peak season, a brilliant display of wildflowers mixes with a lush assemblage of shrubs near the creek, where flowers include lupine, paintbrush, angelica, larkspur and mule ears. Leaving the luxuriant vegetation behind, the trail makes a moderate ascent of a dry hillside until making a turn into a narrow, steep canyon. Climb the slender cleft, twice crossing a seasonal creek, to the wilderness boundary 150 yards below a saddle southwest of Mt. Rose. A short climb leads up to the saddle and a trail junction amid some weather-beaten whitebark

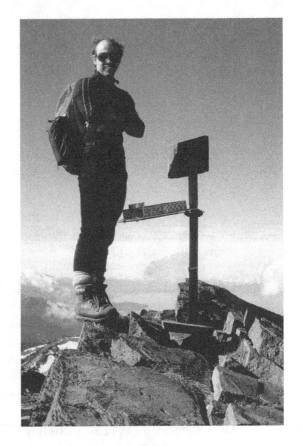

Hiker at the summit of Mt. Rose

pines, 3.6 miles from the trailhead. A sign indicates: MT. ROSE SUMMIT to the right (east) and BIG MEADOWS straight ahead (northwest) toward Bronco Creek.

To reach the summit of Mt. Rose, backpackers should stash their packs near the junction and head through scattered whitebark pines along a narrow ridge toward the gray volcanic mass of Mt. Rose. At the end of the ridge, the grade increases and you begin the first of five switchbacks up the west slope of the peak, views of the surrounding countryside improving with each step. From the switchbacks, the trail makes an ascending traverse around to the northwest side of the mountain, where low-growing alpine plants soon replace the stunted pines. Another series of switchbacks climbs up the rocky slopes, while the actual summit lies just out of view. As

The Myth of Mt. Rose

The origin of the name Mt. Rose is the subject of some curious stories, the most interesting of which claims that a rose can be seen from Reno in the east-face bowl. In actuality, the peak came by its appellation in far less dramatic fashion, named after an early settler, either a Jacob Rose, who built a lumber mill near Franktown, or a Rose Hickman, a friend of a Washoe City newspaper editor.

you approach what seems to be the top, one more set of three short switchbacks brings you to the summit ridge, from where a short jaunt leads to the top.

Human-made improvements at the summit consist of a trail register and rock walls piled high to restrain the notorious winds that frequent the area. If you happen to arrive under calm conditions, count your blessings. Views are quite impressive in all directions. On extremely clear days you can see north all the way to the Cascade volcanoes of Lassen Peak and Mt. Shasta. On normal days the Sierra Buttes are visible in that same general direction, above and beyond the Little Truckee River reservoirs of Prosser, Boca and Stampede. Lake Tahoe is the preeminent gem, encircled by an impressive ring of peaks, including Pyramid Peak and Mt. Tallac in the Desolation Wilderness and Jobs Peak, Jobs Sister and Freel Peak in the Carson Range. Reno-Sparks and the rest of the Truckee Meadows are clearly visible from the summit as well.

To continue toward Bronco Creek, retrace your steps 1.3 miles back to the trail junction, pick up your backpack, and descend moderately through widely scattered whitebark pines to a small meadow, where the grade temporarily abates.

Warning: The path grows indistinct at the near the end of the meadow, but reappears just before the descent resumes.

You quickly realize the contrast between this trail and the more frequented Mt. Rose Trail. Signs of use are so scarce you may begin to wonder if anyone ever hikes here. As the descent continues, the drop in elevation corresponds to an increase in the distribution of pines. Wind your way down, eventually overlooking the broad, sloping meadow of the upper Bronco Creek drainage. Under forest cover, the trail bends and you quickly reach an inconspicuous, unmarked trail junction 1.25 miles from the saddle. The faint trail to the right heads down to Bronco Creek, crosses, and continues north out of the Mt. Rose Wilderness along a jeep road toward Davis and Big meadows. The left-hand trail is reasonably distinct for another quarter mile, but the tread starts to disappear as you approach Bronco Creek, where, near the edge of the trees, a couple of campsites overlook the stream.

Bronco Creek offers solitude in the midst of a tremendous amount of activity. Less than 10 miles away gamblers are cavorting in North Shore casinos, not to mention the numerous hikers much closer, struggling along the trail to the summit of Mt. Rose. Here in the meadows, however, you should have the run of the basin. The rocky faces of Church Peak and Mt. Rose form a dramatic backdrop for the green meadows lining Bronco Creek. Opportunities for further exploration abound, although trails shown on maps may not appear in their entirety on the ground. Although campsites are primitive, there should be an ample supply of firewood.

POSSIBLE ITINERARY

	Camp	Miles	Elevation Gain
Day 1	Mt. Rose Summit/Bronco Creek	7.45	2300
Day 2	Out	4.85	1295

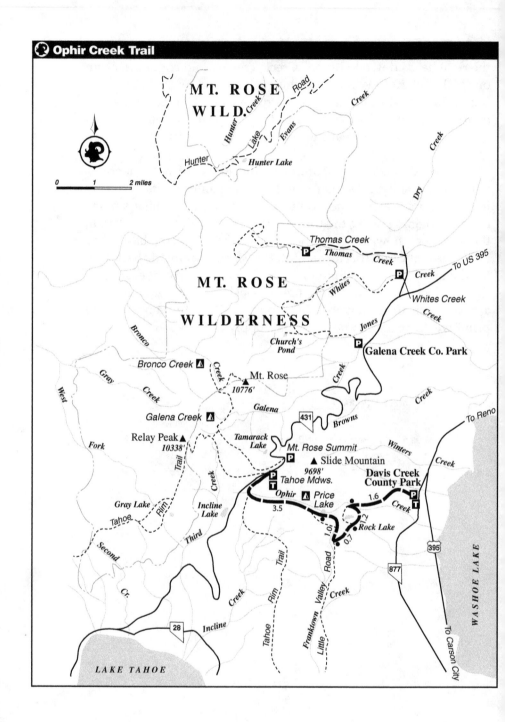

MT. ROSE
WILD.

Hunter Creek

Road

Lake

Evans

Creek

Creek

Hunter

Hunter Lake

Dry

Creek

0   1   2 miles

Thomas Creek

P Thomas

Creek

To US 395

P Creek

MT. ROSE

Whites

Whites Creek

WILDERNESS

Jones

Creek

Church's
Pond

P Galena Creek Co. Park

Bronco

Bronco Creek ▲

Creek

Mt. Rose
▲ 10776'

Creek

Creek

Gray

Creek

West

Galena

Galena Creek ▲

431

Browns

To Reno

Fork

Relay Peak ▲
10338'

Tamarack
Lake

Winters

Creek

Trail

Mt. Rose Summit

P

P ▲ Slide Mountain
9698'

Davis Creek
County Park

Creek

Incline
Lake

T Tahoe Mdws.

P Ophir ▲ Price
Lake
3.5

1.6

P
T

Gray Lake

Rim

1.2

Creek

Tahoe

1.0

Rock Lake

395

Second

Third

0.7

877

Cr.

Creek

Rim

Trail

Franktown Valley Road

Creek

WASHOE LAKE

28 Incline

Tahoe

Little

Creek

To Carson City

LAKE TAHOE

Ophir Creek Trail

RATINGS (1–10)			MILES	ELEVATION GAIN	DAYS	SHUTTLE MILEAGE
Scenery	Solitude	Difficulty				
7	8	8	8	3900	2	27

AREA Carson Range

MAPS USGS - *Washoe City, Mt. Rose*

USUALLY OPEN Early July to mid-October

BEST Mid-July to mid-August

PERMITS None

CONTACT Carson Ranger District (775) 885-6000

SPECIAL ATTRACTIONS Geology, lakes, wildflowers

PROBLEMS Few campsites

HOW TO GET THERE *START:* From U.S. 395, approximately 15 miles south of Reno and 10 miles north of Carson City, turn west following signs for DAVIS CREEK PARK, BOWERS MANSION. Follow S.R. 429, also referred to as Old Highway 395, 0.4 mile to the entrance into Davis Creek Park. Drive through the park, quickly past the equestrian trailhead on the left, and follow the paved access road to the trailhead parking area near a concrete block restroom, complete with flush toilets and running water.

END: Follow S.R. 431, also known as the Mt. Rose Highway, to the Tahoe Meadows trailhead, 0.7 miles west of Mt. Rose Summit and 7.3 miles east of the junction with S.R. 28, which is in Incline Village. Parking is available in a lot on the south shoulder, or down a short access road near a building with flush toilets and running water.

INTRODUCTION Although the Ophir Creek Trail does not enjoy wilderness protection from nearby Mt. Rose Wilderness, this trip offers an abundance of positive attributes, including two small but scenic lakes, a beautiful, 2-mile-long subalpine meadow, tumbling Ophir Creek, and the evidence of a major geological catastrophe.

Mark Twain, astute observer that he was, described the east flank of the Carson Range in *Roughing It,* his chronicle of life in the Far West:

> The mountains are very high and steep about Carson, Eagle and Washoe Valleys—very high and very steep, and so when the snow gets to melting off fast in the spring and the warm surface earth begins to moisten and soften, the disastrous landslides commence. The reader cannot know what a landslide is unless he has lived in that country and seen the whole side of a mountain taken off some fine morning and deposited down in the valley, leaving a vast, treeless, unsightly scar upon the mountain's front to keep the circumstances fresh in his memory all the years that he may go on living within seventy miles of that place.

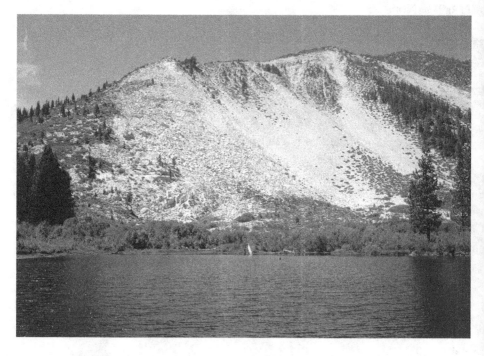

Price Lake and Slide Mountain

Twain's colorful account of history repeated itself most recently in the spring of 1983, when an entire flank of appropriately named Slide Mountain, saturated with meltwater from the thawing winter snows, broke loose and plunged into the canyon of Ophir Creek, instantly displacing the waters of Lower Price Lake. The snow-soaked debris merged with the water from the lake, forming a semi-liquid mass, which roared down the canyon with lightning quickness, consuming everything in its path and reaching the floor of Washoe Valley in a matter of seconds. One death occurred, several homes were destroyed, and acres and acres of debris were spread across the valley, spilling across U.S. 395 and closing the main arterial between Reno and Carson City. As a result of this enormous slide, Lower Price Lake vanished, Upper Price Lake shrank, and the canyon of Ophir Creek was visibly altered. From several spots along the Ophir Creek Trail, hikers can witness the effects of the disaster, although nature has done a lot of healing since 1983.

DESCRIPTION From the trailhead, you hike on wide, sandy tread past sagebrush and manzanita under a light forest of Jeffrey pine, quickly crossing a short, wooden bridge over a tiny seasonal creek and following signs marked OPHIR CREEK TRAIL. Soon, you start to climb more steeply on single-track trail, coming to a junction with the equestrian trail. Beyond the junction, the moderate to moderately steep climb continues up the hillside, occasionally switchbacking across the slope. Along the way are occasional views out to Washoe Lake and Valley. A little over a mile from the trailhead, you come above the deep declivity of Ophir Creek and peer down into the massively eroded, narrow, V-shaped channel. The scoured slope on the opposite side reveals how high the debris from the 1983 slide tore away at the canyon wall.

Away from the viewpoint, you continue the climb through a light forest of Jeffrey pines and scattered shrubs, veering slightly away from the creek for awhile until reaching the edge of a rock-filled vale, where a 4x4 post offers directions for OPHIR CREEK ahead and DAVIS CREEK PARK behind. Nearby, a primitive campsite is just off the trail. Breaking out of the forest, you angle across a boulder-strewn channel to a ford of Ophir Creek, 1.6 miles from the trailhead. Usually an easy boulder-hop, this ford may be difficult in early season. Up the rocky drainage is a good view of Slide Mountain, the source of all these boulders.

Side Trip to Rock Lake: At the far side of the creek channel, a faint, unmarked path veers away from the main trail toward Rock Lake. A short climb leads to the top of a rise, where the trail bends sharply west and drops to a flat, the site of an old cabin. From the flat you climb steeply through dense forest and then even more steeply up a boulder-covered hillside to the crest of a hill, where the path mercifully levels. Rock Lake lies just a short distance beyond, 0.4 mile from the Ophir Creek Trail.

Well-named, Rock Lake reposes in a talus-filled basin, the rocky terrain interrupted only by a small grassy patch along the northwest shore, near a lone campsite. Lily pads cover the surface of the lake, while Jeffrey pines and white firs ring the shoreline. The shallow lake diminishes in size as the summer progresses, and, as the park brochure warns, "don't expect the fishing to be good." **End of Side Trip**

Rather than backtracking, you can regain the Ophir Creek Trail by locating a more distinct trail near the grassy patch on the northwest side of the lake. After a brief level stretch, the trail ascends the manzanita-covered hillside at the east edge of the basin. The grade eases at the top of a rise and then makes a short descent through Jeffrey pines to a signed junction with the main trail, 0.4 mile from the lake.

From the indistinct junction with the faint trail to Rock Lake, the Ophir Creek Trail descends around a forested ridge above the south side of the creek. Where the trail bends back to the west and starts to climb again, you encounter an old road where an old wooden sign marked OPHIR CREEK TR 2007 and a newer 4x4 post helps to keep you on the right path. A stiff climb brings you to the signed junction with the lateral to Rock Lake at 2.75 miles.

A steep, winding climb leads away from the junction through moderate forest cover to the crest of a sub-ridge, where scattered forest, boulders and rock outcroppings provide some variety to the surroundings. Easy hiking on sandy tread leads you across this crest and down to a signed junction with the Little Valley Road, 3.5 miles from the trailhead.

Turn north onto the road, make an initial climb, and then traverse across the slope with good views of Rock Lake below and to the east of Washoe Lake and Valley. After 0.5 mile, you come to another signed junction, where the single-track Ophir Creek Trail bends sharply uphill. Stay on the road for a short distance, heading toward Ophir Creek. Just before the creek is a diversion ditch with a faint path alongside, which parallels the ditch to the outlet of Upper Price Lake. You can elect to follow this path, or remain on the road to a ford of the creek and then head upstream to the lake. Whichever way is chosen, you reach the outlet of Upper Price Lake, 4.5 miles from the trailhead.

Upper Price Lake may be just a remnant of its former self but is still with us, unlike Lower Price Lake, which was completely displaced by debris from the 1983 slide. Inexplicably, the lower lake still appears on the USGS *Washoe City* quadrangle, despite the map's publication date of 1994, more than 10 years after the event. From the picturesque beauty of Upper Price Lake, not being able to enjoy its twin as well seems a shame. Steep slopes plunge into the icy blue waters of Upper Price Lake, not nearly as deep after the slide. The upper canyon forms a sublime backdrop to the serene lake. Campsites are found on the north side of the creek, which means you'll have to carefully negotiate your way across the diversion structure as well as the creek, provided you didn't ford the creek at the road.

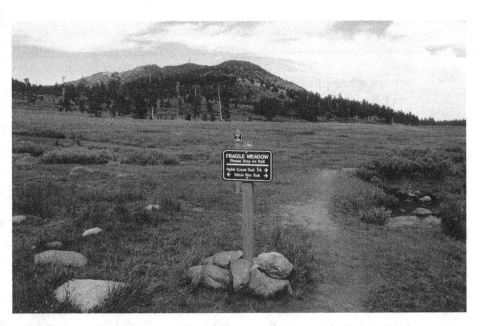

Sign in Tahoe Meadows

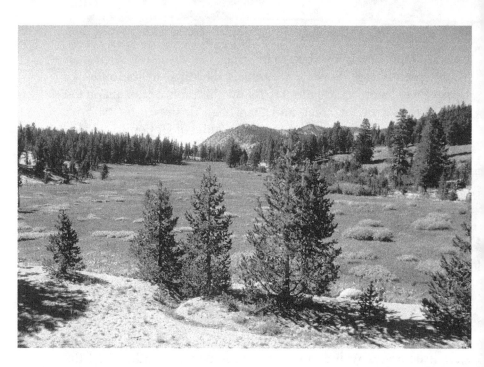

Tahoe Meadows

To continue toward Tahoe Meadows, follow the path on the south side of the lake on a steep ascent across the hillside through a mixed forest of Jeffrey pines, white firs, mountain hemlocks and western white pines. After 0.5 mile of climbing, you rejoin the Ophir Creek Trail. From the junction, the path proceeds up the canyon, crossing a pair of lushly vegetated side streams along the way. The next section of trail has good views, as you alternate through scattered forest and pockets of verdant meadow that through midsummer are filled with a profusion of wildflowers.

A stiff climb takes you back into the moderate cover of a lodgepole-pine forest, as the course of the Ophir Creek Trail stays well into the trees, away from both the creek and Tahoe Meadows. Eventually, easier hiking greets you near the upper end of the trail. After you skirt a small, flower-edged meadow, you come to a twin-tracked jeep road on your left, and after another 0.2 mile reach the junction with the Tahoe Rim Trail, 7 miles from the trailhead. You come to another junction, 0.3 mile farther, between the continuation of the old roadbed heading toward the Mt. Rose Highway and the newly built section of the TRT angling north towards the trailhead.

Remaining on the TRT, you quickly break out of the trees, hop across gurgling Ophir Creek, and then begin a mild ascent across the green expanse of verdant Tahoe Meadows. Backdropped nicely by Slide Mountain, Tahoe Meadows is one of the most scenic sub-alpine meadows in the northern Sierra, despite the presence of a state highway near the fringe. Early season hikers will enjoy a wide range of wildflowers, although the ground can be quite boggy then. Species you can expect to enjoy include buttercup, shooting star, penstemon, elephant head, marsh marigold, paintbrush and large-leaved aven. All too soon, you draw near to the Mt. Rose Highway and stride just below the busy thoroughfare for the last quarter mile to the Tahoe Meadows trailhead.

POSSIBLE ITINERARY

	Camp	Miles	Elevation Gain
Day 1	Upper Price Lake	4.5	2300
Day 2	Out	3.5	1600

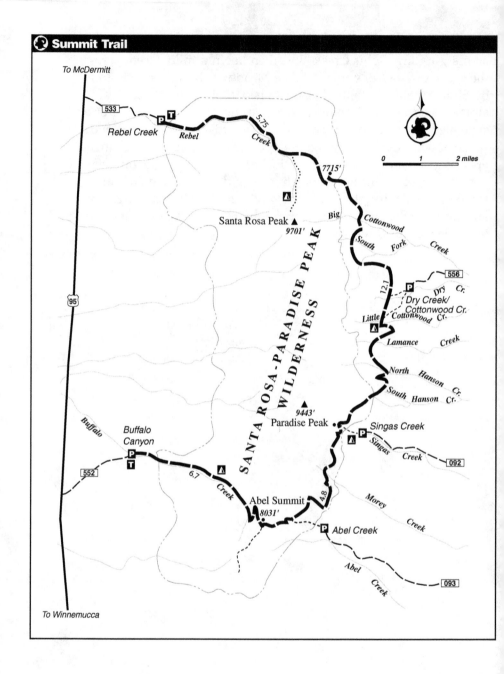

To McDermitt

533

Rebel Creek

Rebel

Creek

5.75

7715'

Santa Rosa Peak ▲
9701'

Big

Cottonwood

South   Fork   Creek

556

95

12.1

Dry   Cr.

Dry Creek/
Cottonwood Cr.
Little   Cottonwood   Cr.

Lamance   Creek

North   Hanson   Cr.

South   Hanson   Cr.

9443'
Paradise Peak

Buffalo
Canyon

Buffalo

Singas Creek

092

Singas   Creek

552

6.7

Creek

4.8

Morey   Creek

Abel Summit
8031'

Abel Creek

Abel   Creek

093

To Winnemucca

4 Summit Trail

RATINGS (1–10)			MILES	ELEVATION GAIN	DAYS	SHUTTLE MILEAGE
Scenery	Solitude	Difficulty				
9	10	9	30	7125	3–4	12

AREA Santa Rosa Range

MAPS USGS-*Santa Rosa Peak, Five Fingers, Adorno Ranch;*
USFS-*Santa Rosa-Paradise Peak Wilderness*

USUALLY OPEN Late June to November

BEST Late June-Early July, October

PERMITS None

CONTACT Winnemucca Ranger District (775) 623-5025

SPECIAL ATTRACTIONS Views, wildflowers, autumn color

PROBLEMS Poor campsites, route finding

HOW TO GET THERE *START:* To reach the north trailhead, follow U.S. 95 north from Winnemucca for 46.5 miles to FS Road 553, signed N. REBEL CREEK ROAD. Head up the well-graded gravel road across grassy fields to an intersection, 0.8 mile from the highway. Follow the less traveled, two-tracked road toward the mountains, following a fence line to a closed gate at 1.4 miles. Continue past the gate into the drainage of Rebel Creek, crossing the stream four times before reaching the end of the road near a grove of cottonwoods, where primitive but shady campsites are nearby.

END: To reach the south trailhead, follow U.S. 95 north from Winnemucca for 36.25 miles to FS Road 552, signed BUFFALO CANYON ROAD. Past a corral, follow the gravel road on a diagonal approach to the mountains and the narrow cleft of Buffalo Canyon. Cross the creek at 2.2 miles and continue for another 0.1 mile to the end of the

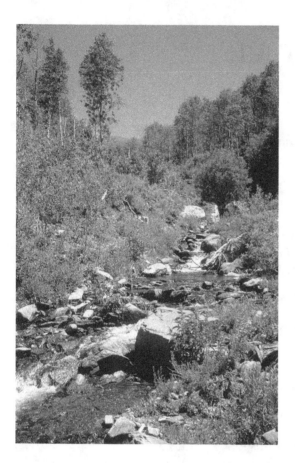

A tumbling creek in Buffalo Canyon, Santa Rosa Range

road, where limited parking is available for just a few vehicles.

INTRODUCTION The Santa Rosa-Paradise Peak Wilderness could be a backpacker's worst nightmare for those unaccustomed to primitive conditions: access roads are rough, the low-elevation approach is blisteringly hot and shadeless in summer, trails are generally unmarked and some sections are indistinct, badly overgrown, or gone altogether. Developed campsites are virtually non-existent, and the range boasts not a single lake. So why would anyone in their right mind consider a backpack into the Santa Rosa Mountains? For starters, how about unparalleled vistas, spectacular wildflower displays, and nearly guaranteed solitude? In addition, the Santa Rosas boast some of the most luxuriant vegetation of any range in the state, thanks to a number of tumbling streams and sweeping basins blessed with ample groundwater. Several of those streams and basins are carpeted with extensive aspen groves, creating a colorful swath of green in summer and a brilliant display of gold in autumn. Early- to midsummer wildflower displays are as fine as any in the state. With such verdant slopes rimmed by rugged granite peaks, the area is more reminiscent of the Rockies than of a typical Great Basin range.

Although many of the short trails leading into the range from a number of trailheads sprinkled on both the west and east sides are suitable for novices on dayhikes, a backpack of the entire Summit Trail is for experienced backcountry travelers only. The poor state of the trail, particularly the stretch outside of the wilderness on the northeast side, requires that backpackers be in good condition and have well-developed route finding skills.

DESCRIPTION The Rebel Creek section of the Summit Trail begins above the north bank of the tumbling, cottonwood-lined stream through a canyon covered with sagebrush, cheat grass and scattered wildflowers.

Warning: Watch for rattlesnakes and ticks, especially in the lower elevations of Rebel Creek and Buffalo Creek canyons.

Phyllite outcroppings add character to the narrow, V-shaped gash. You cross the wilderness boundary 0.5 mile into the hike.

Continue alongside the winding, tumbling creek up the canyon through wild rose, elderberry, cottonwood and the occasional aspen, into the cleft of a large side canyon. Angle across this canyon, cross a diminutive rivulet, and follow the trail back into the main canyon of Rebel Creek, where views up the deep gorge improve with each step.

You skirt another side canyon and follow an old fenceline above the serpentine creek, across a small meadow. Where the canyon narrows, the trail climbs high above the stream to avoid heavy brush and steep cliffs. Thick foliage greets you as you cross a small stream, followed by a descent toward the creek along another fenceline. Eventually, you pass through an open gate to the right and drop down to the north branch of Rebel Creek, 3 miles from the trailhead.

From the crossing, follow the path above the creek into the narrow, steep canyon, where quaking aspens carpet the far hillside. Continue on a moderate ascent until the trail seemingly dead-ends in a tangle of thick brush. Although virtually nonexistent, the trail actually drops to a crossing of the creek and then ascends the far side, where the route becomes distinct again near another pocket of aspens. You climb high above the creek with the aid of a couple of switchbacks and then bend around toward the south up a steep, aspen-choked section of the upper canyon, where dramatic, gray-colored cliffs rise above the stream on the far side.

The ascent continues as you cross the creek near a shady grove of aspen, where the canyon bends east again. Eventually, you climb out of the narrow canyon into less severe topography, where the massive west face of Santa Rosa Peak springs into view. A steep ridge of rugged-looking granite runs along the north ridge of the peak toward the 9,701-foot summit, forming the east edge of a basin that rivals any mountainous area in the state for alpine beauty. Below the peak, the basin is blanketed with what has to be one of the largest stands of aspen in the Great Basin.

The upper basin is a prime area for further explorations as springs and creeks provide abundant water and, although developed sites are virtually nonexistent, potential campsites are plentiful. Santa Rosa Peak should supply a worthy challenge for peak baggers, and the serious mountaineer may find a technical route or two up the sheer granite wall.

Newly constructed trail continues up the creek to the slope below the crest. A final climb leads you across the hillside to the top of the ridge, 5.75 miles from the trailhead. From this vantage, you have a fine view down the east side into the Cottonwood Creek basin and out to Paradise Valley.

Warning: The next section of trail presents the greatest route-finding difficulties along the entire route. Although the terrain is mostly open through this stretch, allowing you to gain your bearings easily, the tread virtually disappears in spots, making sections more of a cross-country route than a bona fide trail.

You drop from the crest, uneventfully crossing the unmarked wilderness boundary after 0.5 mile, and follow Big Cottonwood Creek on a stiff 2-mile descent, losing 1750 vertical feet in the process. Eventually, the route veers away from Big Cottonwood Creek, as you begin a mildly rising traverse into and around the basin of South Fork Cottonwood Creek, hopping across numerous seasonal branches along the way. At 4.75 miles from the trailhead, you reach a saddle on the ridge that divides the South Fork and Dry Creek drainages.

From the saddle, you descend a vanishing path that angles across a sagebrush-carpeted hillside. After a 0.9-mile descent, you reach the jeep road from the Dry Creek trailhead, 5.7 miles from the trailhead, and turn sharply uphill to follow this road on a stiff ascent above the canyon of Dry Creek. After 0.5 mile of steep climbing, the road bends and crosses the upper part of the creek in a swath of aspen. Nearby, a primitive campsite affords a viable option

Paradise Valley

In 1863 a group of miners crossed the Santa Rosas from the west into a lush valley at the eastern base of the range. Apparently quite impressed with the sight, one of the prospectors, W.B. Huff, exclaimed, "What a paradise!" and forevermore the glen was known as Paradise Valley, an appropriate name for the productive agricultural area it eventually became.

for overnighters, but the stream at this elevation is a dependable water source only in early summer.

Beyond Dry Creek, the road rises sharply to a saddle and then drops steeply to a junction near 6450 feet with the road descending to the Little Cottonwood Creek trailhead, 6.6 miles from the Rebel Creek trailhead. Turn west at the junction and begin a traverse around the Cottonwood Creek basin, stepping across a couple of seasonal tributaries before crossing the main branch. Away from the creek, you continue up the side of the canyon without the aid of a trail to a major saddle, directly west of a rocky knob labeled 6537-T on the USGS *Santa Rosa Peak* quadrangle.

A short, gentle climb to the west up a hillside should take you to a fairly distinct path that makes an arcing traverse across the basin holding Lamance and North Fork Hanson creeks. Soon, you reach an unsigned junction with a single-track trail descending the course of the Lamance Creek jeep road, 8.25 miles from the trailhead.

Except where lush vegetation lines the creeks and their numerous tributaries, you traverse across mostly open slopes, accompanied by excellent views of Paradise Valley and the series of ranges in the eastern distance. Beyond the last tributary, a brief ascent leads up to a broad saddle on the ridge separating the North and South Forks of Hanson Creek.

Leaving the saddle, you pass below some rocky cliffs and make a steady climb above the South Fork canyon, utilizing a pair of switchbacks on the way to the next high point along the ridge dividing the Hanson and Singas Creek basins. You continue to enjoy excellent views of Paradise Valley and of the distant ranges to the east, as well as the rugged topography along the east front of the Santa Rosa Range.

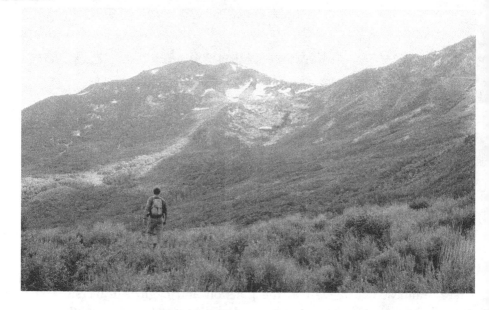

East side of the Santa Rosa Range

A moderate descent leads you down into alternating realms of sagebrush-covered slopes and lush vegetation near the numerous stream channels that feed Singas Creek. Eventually a mild-to-moderate ascent leads through similar terrain to the main channel, followed in 0.2 mile by the unmarked and rather obscure junction with the Singas Creek Trail. From this junction, a 0.4-mile descent leads steeply down to the Singas Creek trailhead, 12.5 miles from the trailhead.

> **Tip:** *With campsites at a premium, you may want to take advantage of the spot near the Singas Creek trailhead, where a small flat next to the creek provides an adequate campsite.*

From the unmarked Singas Creek junction, continue on a gently ascending grade across the basin beneath tall aspens and through lush foliage. Along the way, you cross a pair of seasonal rivulets bordered by moss-covered rocks. Occasionally, the path breaks out into the open, allowing fine views of Paradise Valley below, but when you reach the top of a sagebrush-covered ridge, the vista of the valley and the Singas Creek basin below you, as well as a parade of distant ranges to the east, becomes expansive.

From this aerie, you continue a traverse of drier slopes harboring sagebrush, snowberry and scattered lupines, until a short descent leads you into the Morrey Creek drainage. Hop seasonal streams flanked by groves of aspen, over to the willow-lined main channel of the creek, where wildflowers such as paintbrush and bluebells abound.

Quickly climb out of the drainage and begin an extended descent around the protruding southeast ridge of Singas Peak. You pass through alternating stretches of lush vegetation and open slopes of sagebrush and grasses on the decline around the nose of the ridge and into the Abel Creek basin. Commanding views of Paradise Valley and the distant mountain ranges are virtually continuous.

Across the Abel Creek basin, the Summit Trail follows a horseshoe bend below the open slopes on the south side of Singas Peak. Along the way, you traverse seasonal streams where aspens and willows thrive in the moist soil. Eventually, you follow a short descent into a dense swath of foliage surrounding an upper tributary of Abel Creek. The path may be difficult to follow through this area, but the route continues over the top of a rock-and-wire dam, built for who knows what purpose. Beyond this curious improvement, you climb up to the top of a ridge covered with boulders and mountain mahogany. From this height, the indistinct trail is easily lost in a tangle of brush and small trees before you reach Abel Creek. From the creek, a steep ascent leads to the top of another rise and a junction with the path from the Abel Creek trailhead, 4 miles from the Singas Creek junction.

Beyond the junction, your climb continues toward the ridge-crest. About 30 yards from the actual top, you encounter another junction with a faint path headed southwest along the crest of the range. Veer to the right at this junction and quickly reach Abel Summit, where the views become even more impressive, 4.8 miles from the Singas junction.

Thick brush greets you on the west side of Abel Summit, as you descend steeply with the aid of a pair of long-legged switchbacks. Eventually the grade eases a bit, as you follow the trail down to a meadow. Past the meadow, the trail crosses nascent Buffalo Creek several times while descending through alternating sections of aspen groves, meadows, sagebrush and wildflowers. You hop across the stream to the south bank and continue the descent down the gorge.

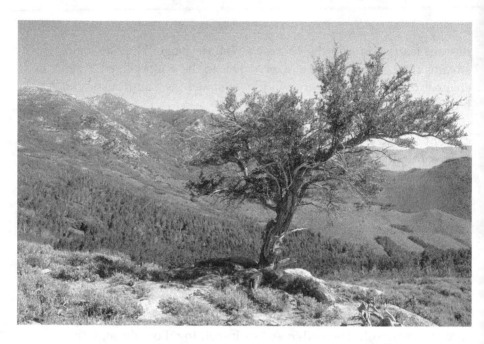

Mountain mahogany tree in Singas Basin, Santa Rosa Range

In and out of thick brush, aspens and cottonwoods, you step over a side stream and make your way down to the next crossing of Buffalo Creek. Just beyond the stream crossing you pass through a flat covered with aspens, cross a lushly lined side stream and come to an even larger flat of mature aspens, affording welcome shade on a hot day.

After a switchback, a steeper descent leads you away from the stream for a spell before the path returns to cross the creek once more. The grade eases as you reach another meadow surrounded by aspen, but a steep descent resumes beyond the meadow, as you pass through open terrain before heading into young aspens above the south bank of the stream and then sagebrush-covered slopes. Soon you reach a large meadow near an aspen grove.

> **Warning:** *Under most circumstances, this meadow would provide some decent campsites. Unfortunately, cattle grazing is permitted within Santa Rosa Wilderness, and if you happen to visit Buffalo Creek Canyon after the cattle have been here, the numerous cow pies here may be sufficient deterrent to choosing this area for a campsite.*

You hop across the stream once more, which in early summer is lined with a lush assortment of wildflowers, including lupine, columbine and monkey flower. Continuing down the narrowing canyon, the trail veers away from the creek for a spell. The vegetation in the lower canyon includes willows, wild rose and aspen along the creek, with mountain mahogany and an occasional limber pine dotting the upper slopes.

After another stream crossing, you continue the descent into the lower canyon, where large outcroppings of phyllite separate Buffalo Creek into two major tributary streams. The trail descends more steeply, past cliffs down to another crossing of the stream, on moss-covered boulders. The last of the aspens are seen in a marshy area below a talus side, as your progress propels you down across sagebrush-covered slopes and past a side canyon.

A switchback leads you to yet another crossing of Buffalo Creek, followed by a winding descent along the tumbling stream, which twists through the serpentine canyon. One final creek crossing leads you to an old roadbed on the north side of the canyon, which you follow past the signed wilderness boundary to a series of narrow benches above the creek. After the benches, you leave the national forest at a fence and soon come to the Buffalo Canyon trailhead and the conclusion of your journey.

POSSIBLE ITINERARY

	Camp	Miles	Elevation Gain
Day 1	Upper Rebel Creek	5.0	2650
Day 2	Singas Creek Trailhead	13.0	2825
Day 3	Out	11.5	1725

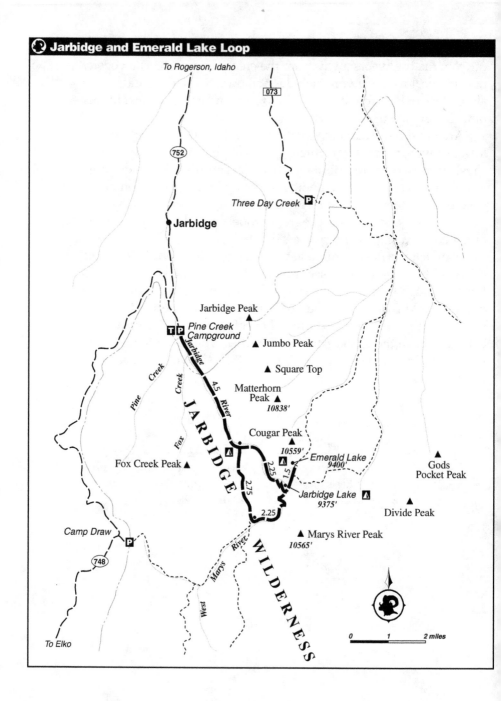

To Rogerson, Idaho

073

752

Three Day Creek 🅿

● Jarbidge

Jarbidge Peak
▲

🅣🅟 Pine Creek
Campground

▲ Jumbo Peak

▲ Square Top

Pine Creek

Fox Creek

Jarbidge River

4.5

Matterhorn
Peak ▲
10838'

J A R B I D G E

Cougar Peak
▲ *10559'*

△ Emerald Lake
9400'

Fox Creek Peak ▲

△

2.25

1.5

2.75

Jarbidge Lake △
9375'

2.25

▲ Marys River Peak
10565'

Gods
Pocket Peak
▲

Divide Peak
▲

Camp Draw
🅟

748

Marys River

West Marys River

W I L D E R N E S S

To Elko

0   1   2 miles

5 Jarbidge and Emerald Lake Loop

RATINGS (1–10)			MILES	ELEVATION GAIN	DAYS	SHUTTLE MILEAGE
Scenery	Solitude	Difficulty				
8	8	6	20	5050	2–4	N/A

AREA Jarbidge Mountains

MAPS USGS-*Jarbidge South, Gods Pocket Peak*; USFS-*Jarbidge Wilderness Map*

USUALLY OPEN Late June to Early October

BEST July

PERMITS None

CONTACT Humboldt National Forest (775) 752-3357

SPECIAL ATTRACTIONS Scenic river canyon, two subalpine lakes, wildflowers, solitude

PROBLEMS Rough sections of trail in first 2.5 miles, difficult fords in high water

HOW TO GET THERE From U.S. 93, 86 miles north of Wells, Nev., and 30 miles south of Twin Falls, Idaho, turn west in the tiny burg of Rogerson, Idaho, onto the Rogerson-Three Creek Road. After approximately 47 miles the paved road turns to gravel. Just before the tiny community of Murphy's Hot Springs, the gravel road comes alongside the Jarbidge River, and narrower road follows the serpentine course of the river through a canyon lined with interesting rock formations.

You eventually cross back into Nevada, as the road becomes Elko County Road 752. At 65 miles from Rogerson, you reach the small but thriving community of Jarbidge. If being in the correct time zone is important, set your watch on Mountain Time, as the locals share the same time zone as their closest neighbors, in Idaho.

Drive through Jarbidge and follow the gravel road across the river four times before reaching the turnoff to the trailhead, 1.9 miles from town. Following a sign for PINE CREEK CG and JARBIDGE WILDERNESS, travel down the dirt road for 0.8 mile to the campground. The trailhead is on the main road at the far end of the campground, relocated in 1995 after a massive slide destroyed sections of the road farther up the canyon. The adjacent campground provides a pleasant setting next to the river, with pit toilets, campfire rings and running water.

INTRODUCTION A roaring river, two subalpine lakes, lofty peaks, verdant meadows, and dense forests await the ardent explorer on this loop through the northwest corner of Jarbidge Wilderness. Although lightly used due to the remoteness of the wilderness, the Jarbidge River Trail to Jarbidge and Emerald lakes is perhaps the

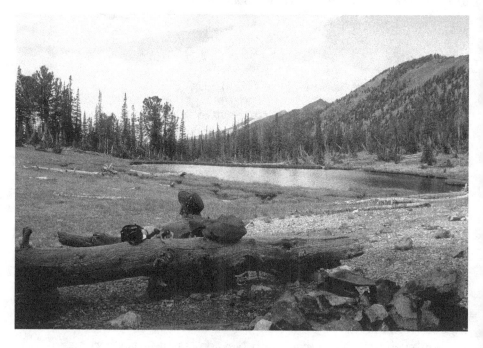

Jarbidge Lake

Jarbidge

The name Jarbidge is a corrupted form of one of two Shoshonean words, either one that means devil or another that comes from a legend about a crater-dwelling giant who wandered Jarbidge canyon capturing natives. The giant would supposedly carry his prey in a basket strapped to his back (making him perhaps the first backpacker in Nevada). Once back at his crater, the giant would then devour his tasty morsels.

most traveled route in the region, and with good reason. With a trailhead accessible by a common sedan, this route is blessed with attractions that any mountain visitor would appreciate.

The beginning of the trail is a testament to the power of nature, as flooding and slides during the spring of 1995 destroyed the road which once led to the old trailhead. High water and soaked debris gouged away sections of the roadbed, resulting in a relocation of the trailhead 1.75 miles downstream, near the Pine Creek Campground. Farther up the drainage, avalanche debris provides a vivid example of what the random forces of the natural world can do.

The two lakes visited by the trail have excellent attributes. Pleasant Jarbidge Lake is a shallow body of water tucked into the head of Jarbidge canyon and surrounded by verdant meadows rimmed by thick forest. The restful ambience provides a grand setting for an afternoon of relaxation while you admire cloud patterns above the lofty summits along the Jarbidge crest. Emerald Lake is a light-green-tinted jewel. Perched below the summit of Cougar Peak and above the deep canyon of the East Fork Jarbidge River, the lakeshore provides commanding views of the surrounding scenery. Sunrises over the eastern range of peaks are particularly stunning.

Early summer provides a colorful array of wildflowers, for which Jarbidge is famous, including arnica, columbine, crimson fireweed, forget-me-not, geranium, Indian paintbrush, lupine, meadowrue, mint, mule ears, pale agoseris, pussytoes, scarlet gilia, sulfur buckwheat, and yarrow. Add in some verdant meadows and dense forests composed of subalpine fir, aspen, limber pine, and whitebark pine, and you have an outstanding complement of flora.

DESCRIPTION Follow the old road through the V-shaped canyon above the east bank of the Jarbidge River amid cottonwoods, aspens, and subalpine fir. Keen eyes will detect the reason for the relocation of the trailhead, as evidence of past slides and flooding is scattered up and down the canyon. You encounter a signed junction with an unmaintained trail ascending the canyon of Fox Creek, 0.6 mile from the campground. Continuing on the Jarbidge River Trail, you cross Fox Creek on a wooden bridge and continue upstream, passing a campsite with picnic table, fire pit and outhouse. A row of large rocks across a remaining section of the old road diverts hikers to a poor stretch of trail above the river. This new section of tread is narrow, brushy, steep in some parts and unstable in others. Late in the season when the water level is down, finding your way along the river may be less of a hassle. During high water you'll be forced to follow this primitive path. Whichever way is chosen, you eventually arrive at the old trailhead below Snowslide Gulch, 2.4 miles from the campground.

Proceed up the canyon, following the track of an old mining road on a climb above the river, flanked by aspens, cottonwoods, subalpine firs, and sporadic whitebark pines. Sagebrush, grasses, and occasional junipers and mountain mahogany trees cover the steep hillsides above. You hop across the stream pouring down Dry Gulch and continue to a crossing of the Jarbidge River at 3.5 miles.

Heading upstream on the west side of the river, you hop over a seasonal stream followed quickly by a crossing of Sawmill Creek on the way to a grassy clearing, where the canyon bends east. In the clearing is a signed junction, at 4.5 miles, with a trail heading south over the ridge and down into the canyon of West Marys River. Your loop trip will return via this trail.

Following signed directions for JARBIDGE RIVER, you head away from the junction to climb more steeply above the river, eventually via a series of switchbacks that lead through dense timber up the narrowing canyon to a river crossing and into meadows on the far side. Open areas filled with wildflowers, grasses, downed timber, and dotted with young subalpine firs suggest that these slopes have been swept by numerous avalanches in the past. After hopping over a few seasonal rivulets, you follow more switchbacks, on a meandering course back under the cover of subalpine firs and then across the diminishing river again. A final series of switchbacks leads you toward the head of the canyon and the gentler terrain of the upper basin. Limber pines and subalpine firs shade the path as you make the easy ascent the last 0.25 mile to lovely Jarbidge Lake, 6.75 miles from the Pine Creek Campground.

Grassy meadows rim the small, deep-blue lake, which nestles in a wide-open basin below sloping hillsides covered with subalpine firs and limber pines. An array of wildflowers adds a splash of color to the lakeshore in early summer. Fine views of the crest abound from the lakeshore, including Matterhorn Peak, at 10,838 feet the highest summit in the Jarbidge Mountains. Fish are absent from these shallow waters—a sure disappointment to any anglers in your group. Backpackers will find mature trees sheltering a few campsites above the south shoreline, and additional sites along the outlet. Since most parties seem to push on toward Emerald Lake, solitude at Jarbidge Lake is a reasonable expectation, whether you plan to camp or just relax for a spell near the placid waters.

Continuing on your journey, the trail arcs around Jarbidge Lake before switchbacking toward the saddle directly southeast of the lake. At the saddle, you reach a three-way junction, where a sign points northeast (uphill) to:

COUGAR MOUNTAIN TRAIL, EMERALD LAKE 2.5

EAST FORK JARBIDGE RIVER 5.3

and south (downhill) to:

CAMP DRAW W. MARYS RIVER TRAIL, W. FORK MARYS RIVER 2.2

76 CREEK DIVIDE 6.9

MARYS RIVER 8.0

Views from the saddle down both the West Marys and Jarbidge rivers are quite dramatic.

From the saddle, a moderate ascent incorporating five switchbacks leads you to the top of the ridge that separates the Jarbidge and East Jarbidge canyons. Amid widely scattered and stunted limber pines, the sweeping vista from impressive Marys River Peak all the way down the East Jarbidge River canyon is quite stunning.

A series of long switchbacks eases you down the steep hillside to a long, descending traverse that passes above a pair of small tarns perched on an open bench and continues to a junction amid dense timber. Following signed directions for EMERALD LAKE, you make a short gentle climb through moderate forest up to the lake, 8.25 miles from the campground.

Emerald Lake, so named for the beautiful green complexion, is a precious gem cradled beneath the red-tinged rock of 10,559-foot

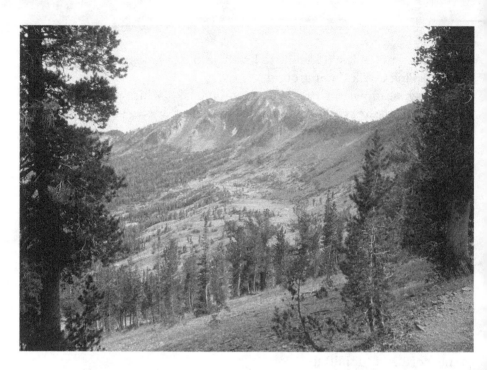

Marys River Peak near Emerald Lake, Jarbidge Mountains

Cougar Peak. Bordered by a horseshoe basin rimmed by jagged cliffs, the lake reposes on a lofty perch above the canyon of the East Fork Jarbidge River, 1800 feet below. Scattered pines adorn the shoreline and wildflowers crown the banks of the inlet and outlet streams. A mild rise above the east shore has campsites, perhaps the best one being above the far end of the lake. Unlike the sterile waters of Jarbidge, Emerald has a healthy population of brook trout. Early mornings at the 9400-foot-high lake can be chilly, but sunrises can be quite spectacular.

From the pleasant surroundings of Emerald Lake, retrace your steps 1.5 miles to the three-way junction in the saddle above Jarbidge Lake. From the saddle, follow Trail No. 019 on a long switchbacking descent across rocky slopes dotted with limber pine and subalpine fir. Farther downslope, the trail alternates between stands of subalpine fir and pockets of grassy meadow, until rabbitbrush and sagebrush become the dominant vegetation near the floor of the canyon.

Eventually, as the trail comes alongside West Marys River, the foliage on either side stands in stark contrast to that on the other.

The north-facing slopes are heavily timbered, while sagebrush and grasses dominate the nearly treeless, south-facing slopes. After a while, near a broad meadow, the trail veers away from the river and reaches a signed junction at the far end, 2.25 miles from the saddle. Nearby, a nice campsite on the east side of the side stream will tempt backpackers seeking overnight accommodations.

At the junction, turn north from the West Marys River Trail and follow moderately graded switchbacks across the grass-and-sage-covered slope. As you gain elevation, a few pines start to appear, and by the time you reach the crest, 1.5 miles later, you find yourself in a sandy saddle surrounded by firs, with filtered views of the Jarbidge crest.

Small pockets of verdant meadow surrounded by thick stands of subalpine fir greet you on the north side of the crest, as the trail plunges you headlong toward the Jarbidge River. Quickly pass the remains of an old cabin near a spring-fed rivulet, where the forest thins just enough to allow a fine view of the crest. Beyond the cabin, steep switchbacks lead across steep cliffs and back into dense forest. The trail follows the tumbling creek down the declivitous canyon through a mixed forest of subalpine fir, limber pine and quaking aspen. You cross the stream twice before reaching the junction with the Jarbidge River Trail, 1.25 miles from the saddle. About 75 yards before the junction, a very pleasant campsite lies next to the stream near a stand of aspens.

From the junction, retrace your steps 4.5 miles down the Jarbidge River Trail to the trailhead at Pine Creek Campground.

POSSIBLE ITINERARY

	Camp	Miles	Elevation Gain
Day 1	Emerald Lake	8.25	3550
Day 2	Jarbidge River	6.5	1400
Day 3	Out	4.5	100

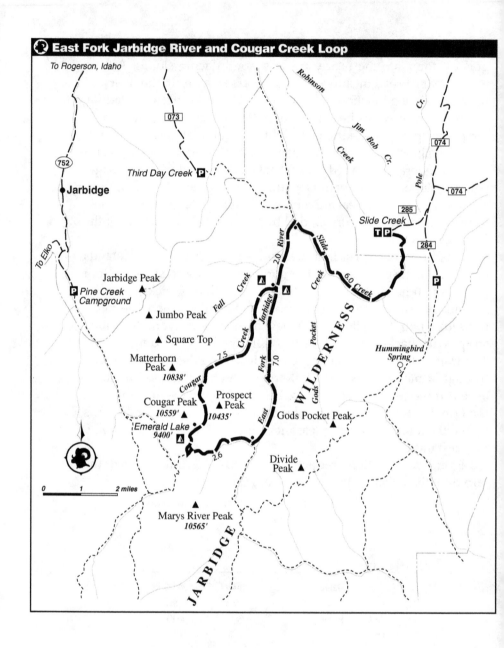

6   East Fork Jarbidge River and Cougar Creek Loop

RATINGS (1–10)			MILES	ELEVATION GAIN	DAYS	SHUTTLE MILEAGE
Scenery	Solitude	Difficulty				
8	9	8	29	5990	4–5	N/A

AREA Jarbidge Mountains

MAPS USGS-*Robinson Peak, Gods Pocket Peak*; USFS-*Jarbidge Wilderness Map*

USUALLY OPEN Late June to mid-October

BEST July

PERMITS None

CONTACT Humboldt Ranger District (775) 738-5171

SPECIAL ATTRACTIONS Wildflowers, views, diverse landscape, solitude, good canyon scenery, Emerald Lake

PROBLEMS Rattlesnakes and heat in lower canyons, difficult stream crossings in early season

HOW TO GET THERE Drive U.S. 93 to the tiny burg of Rogerson, Idaho, approximately 86 miles north of Wells, Nev., and 30 miles south of Twin Falls, Idaho. In Rogerson, head west on the Rogerson-Three Creek Road, following two-lane, paved highway about 36.5 miles to a junction, just a few hundred feet beyond the Three Creek School. Turn left at the junction, following a sign reading POLE CREEK 16.

Head south on gravel road, crossing Pole Creek at 5.5 miles and the Nevada border at 6.5 miles. At 9.5 miles, you cross into Forest Service land and continue on FS Road 074. Proceed to a Y-junction, 14.75 miles from the highway, and veer left following a sign for

CANYON CREEK 6, ELK MOUNTAIN 12, and ONEIL BASIN 14 (the right-hand road reaches the Pole Creek Ranger Station after a mile).

Continue on FS 074 for 1.25 miles to a junction, where FS 074 bends east, and turn onto the rougher surface of FS 284. After 0.25 mile, you reach another junction, where FS 284 continues straight ahead toward the Hummingbird trailhead.

Leaving FS 284, you turn right (south) onto FS 285 and travel 1.1 miles to another Y-junction, passing a couple of lesser roads along the way. Following a sign marked SLIDE CREEK TRAILHEAD, turn left and drive on FS 285A a short distance to the trailhead, which lies in a grove of aspen and subalpine fir, approximately 17.75 miles from the highway.

Scattered around the trailhead area are a few sheltered campsites with running water available from a nearby stream.

INTRODUCTION The East Fork Jarbidge River-Cougar Creek Loop is one of the premier backcountry experiences in the Jarbidge Mountains. The unparalleled scenery is only one of the many rewards found along the loop, which passes through a wide variety of topography. Along the nearly 30-mile journey, backpackers witness high-elevation tablelands with spectacular vistas, roaring streams that course down precipitous canyons, and even a subalpine lake perched majestically below a towering peak.

The plant zones experienced along the route are equally as diverse. The fine assortment of tree species includes aspen, cottonwood, mountain mahogany, juniper, subalpine fir and limber pine. Where trees are absent, open slopes carpeted with grasses and sagebrush are complemented nicely by dramatic vistas. Early summer is graced with a bounty of wildflowers, for which the Jarbidge Mountains are noted, including such varieties as arnica, agoseris, balsamroot, bluebells, columbine, forget-me-not, geranium, lupine, meadowrue, monkey flower, monkshood, paintbrush, shooting star, and yarrow.

Although early summer is the best time to visit for the wildflower displays, this part of the season isn't without hazards. Backpackers must negotiate numerous fords of the East Fork Jarbidge River along the route, as well as crossings of Slide, Cougar and Third Day creeks. If your visit is scheduled for June or early July, check with the Forest Service regarding stream flows before setting out on this loop.

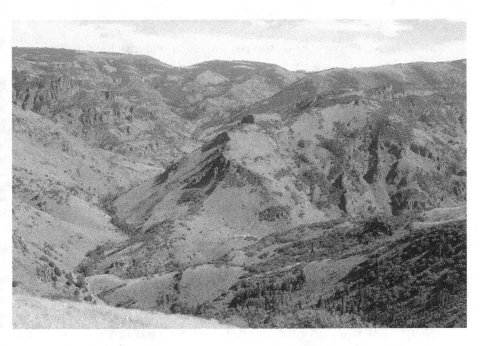

Slide Creek and East Fork Jarbidge River canyons, Jarbidge Mountains

An unwritten rule of the backcountry holds that a good trail is one that starts low, climbs high and then returns downhill to the car. The East Fork Jarbidge River-Cougar Creek Loop fails to meet this criterion, alternately losing and gaining vast sums of elevation over the 29-mile course. Despite the up-and-down nature of the trail, the mountain grandeur along the East Fork Jarbidge River-Cougar Creek loop will satisfy the most critical wilderness enthusiast.

Tip: An extra vehicle would allow you to vary the route somewhat by returning to either the Hummingbird Spring or Third Day Creek trailhead.

DESCRIPTION Pass through sagebrush and grasses as the trail heads east and then southeast along a small tributary down to the main channel of nascent Slide Creek. You follow the course of the tiny rivulet downstream, crossing the signed wilderness boundary around the 0.75-mile mark. Beyond the boundary, the canyon deepens, the volume of water in the creek increases, and the vegetation becomes more profuse. Subalpine fir and aspen, along with various shrubs and flowers, begin to crowd the stream in the narrowing canyon.

Over the next mile, the path leads you across the creek several times—crossings that may prove rather damp in early summer. Through infrequent breaks in the foliage, you gain limited views of the dramatic rock cliffs forming the upper limits of the deep chasm of Slide Creek. Farther down the canyon, the lush riparian vegetation gives way to a drier zone, and where the canyon veers west, mountain mahogany and chokecherry begin to claim the hillsides from the aspen and subalpine fir above.

You continue down the trail, following the course of the serpentine, V-shaped canyon as it bends northwest. At 4 miles from the trailhead, Gods Pocket Creek converges with Slide Creek, having dropped 3000 feet from the upper slopes of Gods Pocket Peak in 3.5 miles. The steady descent continues down the canyon toward the confluence with East Fork Jarbidge River Trail, which you reach at 6 miles and 2155 feet in elevation from the trailhead.

Beyond the junction, the main trail crosses Slide Creek, climbs up a low rise above the far bank, and proceeds upstream along the East Fork, where a smattering of cottonwoods, subalpine fir, mountain mahogany, and junipers dots the hillsides. On the opposite bank, 0.8 mile from the junction, where Fall Creek converges with the river, an unmaintained path heads upstream for nearly a mile, to where it meets and follows the north branch of the creek before climbing to a trailhead on top of Sawmill Ridge. Remaining on the East Fork Trail, you travel another 1.2 miles to the somewhat obscure junction with the Cougar Creek Trail, 8 miles from the trailhead.

Cross the East Fork, where you'll find a fair campsite on the far bank, and begin the ascent of Cougar Creek Canyon, traveling high up the hillside above the stream through juniper, aspen and mahogany. At 0.75 mile from the junction, you cross Cougar Creek and proceed steeply up the east bank amid sagebrush, grasses and wildflowers.

You stay well above the creek for a considerable distance, until the canyon bends southwest and you enter a dense stand of aspens. Before the trail veers away from the creek again, you pass a lone campsite, shaded by subalpine firs. Continuing up the canyon, you arrive at a steep, open slope sprinkled with a few young firs, a good indicator that this hillside has seen an avalanche or two. Your suspicion is confirmed a short distance farther up the trail, where the path slices across an even more extensive avalanche swath. Beyond the snow-swept hillsides, a winding trail incorporating a trio of switchbacks brings you to an old log cabin near a meadow-covered hillside fed by a spring.

Past more avalanched slopes, the trail zigzags up to another old cabin. This structure is in remarkably good shape, housing many artifacts that are also in excellent condition. A short distance farther the trail encounters a spring-fed meadow, which was more than likely the water source for the cabin's occupant.

Nearing the head of the canyon, you make a moderate, zigzagging ascent through limber pines to a pass between Cougar and Prospect peaks, on the ridge separating Cougar Creek from the East Fork. Fine views above Cougar Creek extend to the mountains of Idaho to the north, and down into the deep gorge below Marys River Peak to the south.

A gray, gravel path heads down the backside of the ridge, switchbacking through more limber pines. As you descend, Emerald Lake appears in the basin below. At the bottom of the switchbacks, you reach the upper basin and pass a secluded campsite bordered by some stunted pines. A short, gentle stroll brings you to the northeast shore of Emerald Lake, 7.5 miles from the Slide Creek-East Fork junction.

Emerald Lake, so named for the beautiful green complexion, is a precious gem cradled beneath the red-tinged rock of 10,559-foot Cougar Peak. Bordered by a horseshoe basin of jagged cliffs, the lake reposes on a lofty perch above the canyon of the East Fork Jarbidge River, 1800 feet below. Scattered pines adorn the shoreline and wildflowers crown the banks of the inlet and outlet streams. A mild rise above the east shore holds campsites, perhaps the best one being above the far end of the lake. Unlike the sterile waters of Jarbidge, Emerald has a healthy population of brook trout. Early mornings at the 9400-foot-high lake can be chilly, but sunrises can be quite spectacular.

From the lake, make a mild descent south to a signed three-way junction with the trail coming over the ridge from Jarbidge Lake. Following signed directions for E FORK JARBIDGE RIVER, you proceed straight ahead for a short distance to an inconspicuous, unmarked T-junction: The East Fork Trail actually bends 90 degrees to the left, as a more heavily used path continues straight ahead, reaching an

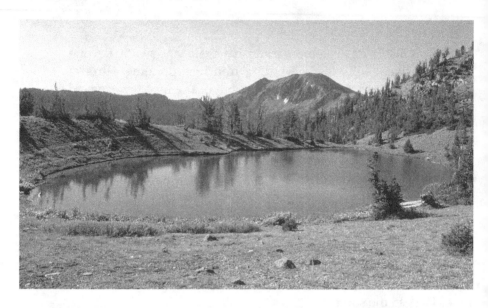

Emerald Lake with Marys River Peak in the distance, Jarbidge Mountains

outfitters camp after 0.75 mile. The junction, possibly marked by a cairn, is easily missed, so pay close attention—if you eventually come to a tarn on a long bench you have missed the turn.

From the primitive junction, the trail descends through small, scattered pines and firs, grasses and wildflowers, past a small open flat surrounded by conifers, where an outfitter operates a seasonal horse camp. A somewhat obscure section of the trail bends sharply away from the flat, headed toward the East Fork canyon. Across a stretch of open terrain, the path becomes distinct again and then starts to descend more steeply toward the gorge, crossing seasonal rivulets and grassy meadows along the way. Sagebrush becomes the principal ground cover as you near the mahogany-lined creek. Paralleling the East Fork Jarbidge River, you pass over numerous side streams bordered by lush foliage, reaching a signed junction with the Camp Creek Trail, 2.6 miles from Emerald Lake.

Another 0.25 mile down the trail, you begin a 3-mile section of relocated trail that differs from what is shown on the USGS map. Avalanches decimated the old section of trail in the bottom of the canyon, so the Forest Service built this newer stretch of trail across the slopes above the river. The relocated trail heads into a side canyon, crosses the diminutive creeklet amid firs, cottonwoods and aspens, and then begins a series of switchbacks up the mahogany-

and juniper-covered hillside. After gaining sufficient elevation, you traverse back into the main canyon and proceed through grasses, sagebrush, and wildflowers past an occasional limber pine and mountain mahogany.

For the next couple of miles, you traverse the east side of the canyon high above the level of the creek, climbing in and out of several side canyons along the way, where you cross small tributaries of the East Fork amid lush riparian vegetation. At the end of the long traverse, a steep descent takes you back down near the river to a connection with the old trail again.

Now on the old trail, you cross a pair of side streams and head downstream, alternating through sagebrush and grasses above the river and cottonwoods and subalpine firs along the bottom of the canyon. Where the trail follows the course of an old roadbed, campsites can be had on a large flat next to the river, near where a use-trail leads to a horsepacker's camp on the opposite side. Just beyond this use-trail, you close your loop at the junction with the Cougar Creek Trail, 7.5 miles from Emerald Lake.

From the junction, retrace your steps 8 miles to the Slide Creek trailhead.

POSSIBLE ITINERARY

	Camp	Miles	Elevation Gain
Day 1	Lower Cougar Creek	8.0	375
Day 2	Emerald Lake	7.5	3320
Day 3	East Fork Jarbidge River	7.0	160
Day 4	Out	6.0	2135

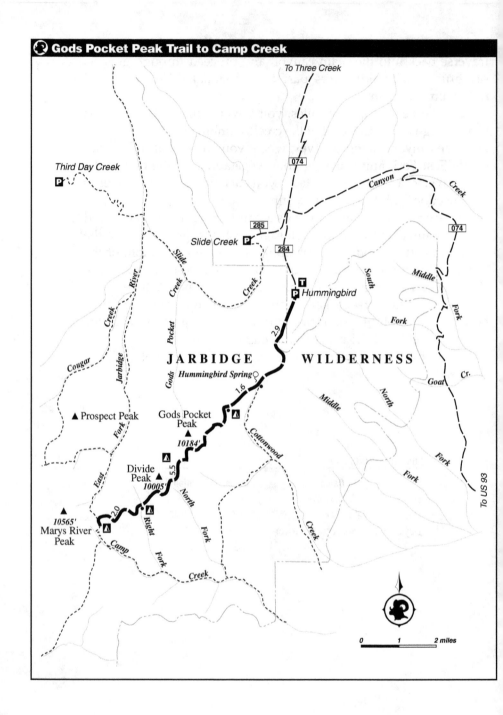

7 Gods Pocket Peak Trail to Camp Creek

RATINGS (1–10)			MILES	ELEVATION GAIN	DAYS	SHUTTLE MILEAGE
Scenery	Solitude	Difficulty				
9	10	5	24	5225	2–4	N/A

AREA Jarbidge Mountains

MAPS USGS-*Goat Creek, Gods Pocket Peak*; USFS-*Jarbidge Wilderness Map*

USUALLY OPEN Late June to Early October

BEST July

PERMITS None

CONTACT Humboldt Ranger District (775) 738-5171

SPECIAL ATTRACTIONS Views, scenery, solitude

PROBLEMS Sheep

HOW TO GET THERE Drive U.S. 93 to the tiny burg of Rogerson, Idaho, approximately 86 miles north of Wells, Nev., and 30 miles south of Twin Falls, Idaho. In Rogerson, head west on the Rogerson-Three Creek Road, following two-lane, paved highway about 36.5 miles to a junction, just a few hundred feet beyond the Three Creek School. Turn left at the junction, following a sign reading POLE CREEK 16.

Head south on gravel road, crossing Pole Creek at 5.5 miles and the Nevada border at 6.5 miles. At 9.5 miles, you cross into Forest Service land and continue on FS Road 074. Proceed to a Y-junction, 14.75 miles from the highway, and veer left following a sign for CANYON CREEK 6, ELK MOUNTAIN 12, and ONEIL BASIN 14 (the right-hand road reaches the Pole Creek Ranger Station after a mile).

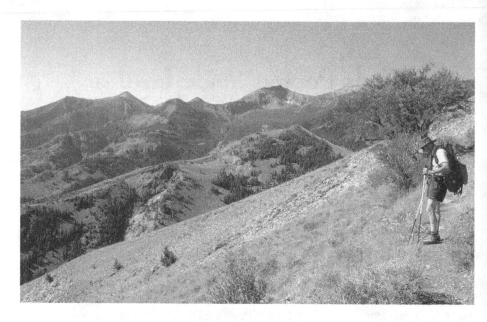

Gods Pocket Peak, Jarbidge Mountains

Continue on FS 074 for 1.25 miles to a junction, where FS 074 bends east, and turn onto the rougher surface of FS 284. After 0.25 mile, you reach another junction, where you continue straight ahead on FS 284 toward the Hummingbird trailhead. You follow a fence 1.1 miles to a junction, where you bear left along an old pole fence for 0.25 mile until the road bends and climbs to its end on top of a broad ridge, about 18.5 miles from the highway. Nearby, shaded by some pines, are a couple of dry campsites.

INTRODUCTION Solitude is a staple of Jarbidge Wilderness, but even horse packers seem to shy away from the Gods Pocket Peak Trail, even though some of the most picturesque scenery in the area is found along this path. From the very beginning, spectacular vistas reign as the chief attributes of the journey, and each step offers more stunning glimpses of the surrounding ranges and canyons. Midway through the trip, a 3-mile traverse on narrow trail clinging to precipitous slopes (perhaps the reason horse packers avoid the trail) offers nearly continuous panoramas of the vast Nevada landscape.

Campsites are few, but so is the demand, and some of them offer excellent aeries from which to take in the views and awake to a spectacular sunrise, although water may be scarce in late season.

The one glaring drawback to the trip is the damage that cattle and sheep have done to the area around Hummingbird Spring. Hooves have totally ravaged the lush meadow surrounding the spring, and one can only imagine how polluted the water may be from the urine and feces of that much stock.

Tip: At a pair of junctions near the end of the trip around Camp Creek, the Gods Pocket Peak Trail connects to three other trails, providing plenty of opportunities for extending the journey into other magnificent areas of the Wilderness. A short car shuttle would enable a lengthy extension through much of Jarbidge Wilderness with a terminus at the Camp Draw, Snowslide, Third Day, or Slide Creek trailheads.

DESCRIPTION The route begins by following the continuation of the road heading south along the crest of a broad, grassy ridge. Scattered limber pines dot the edge of the knoll, and small chips of obsidian testify to the volcanic origin of the range. Proceeding along the ridge, you pass a few campsites providing stunning views across the East Fork Jarbidge River to the Jarbidge Range, including 10,838-foot Matterhorn Peak. Your journey along the crest is briefly interrupted by a stretch of single-track trail, which descends through low sagebrush and grasses to a resumption of the road on a bench.

You briefly enter a pocket of subalpine fir, limber pine and aspen, before breaking into the open at a clearing filled with sagebrush and grasses, where Gods Pocket Peak looms in the near distance. A moderate descent leads to Hummingbird Spring near a broad, sloping meadow, which, depending on the season and amount of visitation by stock, may be a muddy morass of trodden soil. Follow the trail downslope 200 yards from the spring to a signed junction near the creek that flows from the spring, 2.9 miles from the trailhead.

Following signed directions for GODS POCKET PEAK TRAIL, head over the creek, and continue around and over an open hillside. A gradual descent through sagebrush, grasses, and flowers leads into the Cottonwood Creek drainage. As you approach the first ravine, mountain mahoganies, aspens, subalpine firs, and limber pines begin to appear. In an open meadow fringed with firs, the trail passes below a pipe carrying spring water. Beyond the pipe, you cross another seasonal stream and come to aspen-lined Cottonwood

Creek, 4.25 miles from the trailhead. On the far bank, a use-trail leads upstream to a pleasant campsite sheltered by subalpine firs.

You climb steeply away from the creek, across a hillside covered with firs and pines, until the grade eases and the forest thins near a small knoll, where you begin a pleasant, curving traverse over to a saddle. From the saddle, head south from Gods Pocket Peak as the trail dips in and out of minor drainages on a 3.5-mile traverse below the ridge crest. Shortly after the steep slopes of Gods Pocket Peak, you pass a willow-lined channel where a spring sends a narrow trickle across the path. Below steep cliffs, the tread becomes rocky as you proceed through widely scattered limber pines and subalpine firs. Fabulous views abound throughout the traverse, including a vista of the East Humboldt and Ruby Mountain ranges in the distant southwest. The traverse continues in and out of light forest past four seasonal creeks to the top of a minor ridge at 6.75 miles, where a lone campsite reposes in the open grass, surrounded by some conifers. Although campers have to travel a considerable distance back to the stream for water, the views from this grassy perch more than compensate for this inconvenience.

From the minor ridge you head back into light forest and contour over to a lushly vegetated spring in the next canyon. Beyond the spring, the trail ascends more steeply through scattered limber pines to a pass south of Divide Peak, 8.5 miles from the trailhead. Here, at the end of the 3.5-mile traverse, you begin a steep, plunging descent.

Entering thick subalpine fir forest, you leave the vistas behind and follow steep switchbacks, dropping 1250 feet in 1.5 miles to the floor of the canyon of the Right Fork Camp Creek. Campsites along the creek provide a welcome reward for the 10-mile hike.

From the Right Fork Camp Creek, a moderate 1.25-mile ascent takes you out of the Right Fork canyon to the rocky crest of a ridge separating it from the Camp Creek drainage. From there a 0.5-mile descent brings you to a signed junction with Trail No. 200, which provides a 3-mile connector to the East Fork Jarbidge River Trail (see Trip 6, p. 93). The Gods Pocket Peak Trail follows a zigzagging 0.25-mile descent from the junction down to Camp Creek, where backpackers will find a few shady campsites along the creek.

From Camp Creek, you have a few options for further wanderings. More ambitious backpackers can continue on the Gods Pocket

Peak Trail for 1.25 miles to a three-way junction and the start of the Marys River Basin Trail No. 195, which leads southwest to Marys River Basin and a junction with the Marys River Trail No. 018.

POSSIBLE ITINERARY

	Camp	Miles	Elevation Gain
Day 1	6.75-mile Camp	6.75	1050
Day 2	Camp Creek	5.25	1375
Day 3	Out	12.0	2850

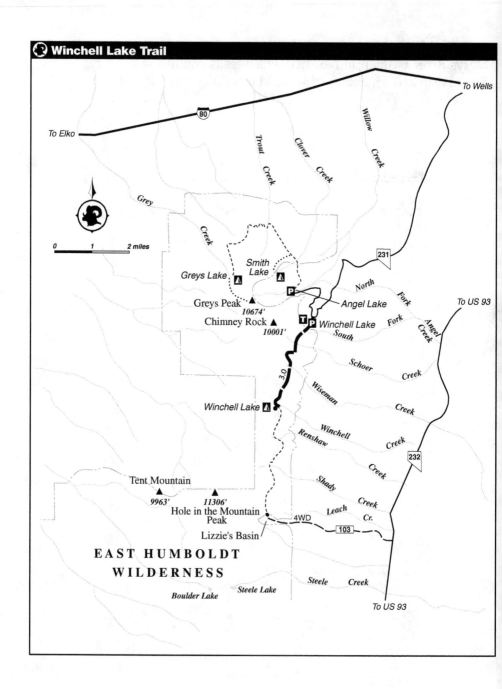

8 Winchell Lake Trail

RATINGS (1–10)			MILES	ELEVATION GAIN	DAYS	SHUTTLE MILEAGE
Scenery	Solitude	Difficulty				
8	9	2	6	1110	2–3	N/A

AREA East Humboldt Mountains

MAPS USGS-*Welcome, Humboldt Peak*; USFS-*Ruby Mountains and East Humboldt Wildernesses*

USUALLY OPEN Early July to mid-October

BEST Mid-July to mid-August

PERMITS None

CONTACT Ruby Mountains Ranger District (775) 752-3357

SPECIAL ATTRACTIONS Winchell Lake, mountain scenery, solitude, foliage

PROBLEMS Infrequently maintained trail, poor campsites

HOW TO GET THERE From Interstate 80, take the WEST WELLS exit, No. 351, turn south onto U.S. 93 and immediately west onto State Route 231, signed ANGEL LAKE. Follow paved road into Forest Service land at 7 miles from the highway, and, 0.3 miles farther, continue past the turnoff to Angel Creek Campground. Soon the road narrows and makes a steep, winding climb up the foothills. At 9.75 miles, in the midst of a hairpin turn, you pass the Winchell Lake trailhead below the far shoulder. Parking for a few vehicles is available just up the road on the right-hand shoulder.

INTRODUCTION The journey to Winchell Lake takes hikers and back-packers into the heart of the east side of remote East Humboldt Wilderness. A distance of 3 miles and a mild 1000-foot elevation gain make for a relatively gentle trip, but despite this ease, the trail sees little use. En route to the lake you'll encounter numerous creeks and rivulets that refresh pockets of lush riparian habitat. The trail provides excellent views of the East Humboldt Mountains from various localities, and lovely subalpine scenery at two lake basins — one along the way and one that holds the lake. A campsite at Winchell Lake offers scenery, solitude, potential for further wanderings, and the opportunity to wake up to an awesome sunrise.

DESCRIPTION The trail, not shown on the USGS map, leads you down from the highway into a lush pocket of shrubs, wildflowers and aspens, and quickly across a seasonal stream. Beyond this rivulet, the foliage diminishes enough to allow views of rugged Chimney Rock above, and the ranchland below. The path climbs and drops through a mixture of vegetation, ranging from aspens, shrubs and flowers to the more common sagebrush-covered slopes. You enter East Humboldt Wilderness just before the crossing of South Fork Angel Creek, a tumbling stream that courses through a verdant

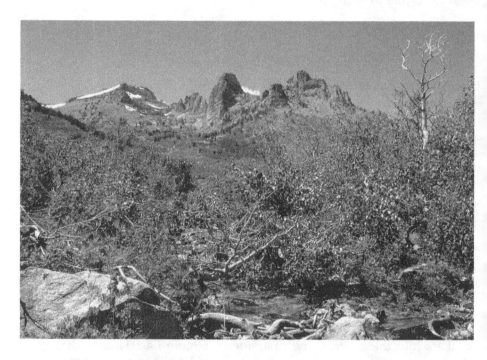

Chimney Rock above Schoer Creek, East Humboldt Range

swath of foliage and flowers, with the rugged cliffs of Chimney Rock presenting a dramatic backdrop. A short distance from the first, you make a second crossing, where almost the entire eastern front of the East Humboldt Mountains is visible, spanning from Chimney Rock in the north to Humboldt Peak in the south.

Away from South Fork Angel Creek, you skirt a grove of mature aspens and pass through the gate of a barbed-wire fence into a grassy field, where the trail becomes indistinct for a bit. More discernible trail quickly appears again as you make a mild climb, followed by a descent to Schoer Creek, 0.9 mile from the trailhead.

You cross the brush-choked stream, wind around a hillside and descend to a dry streambed. The grade of the trail moderates as you make a protracted traverse across slopes covered with tobacco brush and aspen. As you traverse, you realize that some four-footed beasts have preceded your visit: beavers have constructed a number of ponds on the hillside below, and cattle have left their calling cards along the path. The nearly level grade lasts for about 0.75 mile before a steeper descent leads you down to the next creek. Just before the stream you see the results of some of that beaver activity up close, as the trail skirts one of their ponds, allowing a very good look at beaver habitat. A good dirt path leads away from the beaver pond to a curious junction, where one branch of the trail continues straight ahead and the other turns 90 degrees to the right.

Take the right-hand path and climb uphill for about 75 yards before veering south again. A mildly undulating trail leads to a climb into Wiseman Basin, a spectacular, horseshoe-shaped amphitheater of rugged cliffs, where a cascade tumbles down the sheer rock face above. As the path wanders across the floor of the picturesque basin, you expect to meet Wiseman Creek at some point, but the stream follows a subterranean path below the marshy ground before emerging in the canyon farther downstream. If you have the time, Wiseman Basin is certainly worthy of further exploration.

From the basin, you ascend a sagebrush-covered hillside, head back into tobacco brush on an up-and-down course, and then climb in earnest past a seasonal stream to a pair of switchbacks that lead you up the slope to the shore of Winchell Lake, 3 miles from the trailhead.

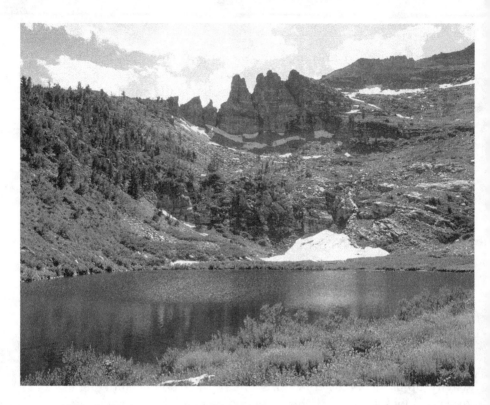

Winchell Lake, East Humboldt Range

Winchell Lake, at 8570 feet, rests in another dramatic basin, with green, sloping hillsides rising up to steep, jagged peaks, where the crest reaches heights over 10,000 feet in less than a mile from the lakeshore. Three triangular spires above the inlet form an impressive backdrop to the dark waters of the lake. Verdant meadows at the far end blend into dense green foliage around the rest of the shoreline. A smattering of limber pines dots the southwest slopes in the otherwise open basin, which plays host to a wide range of vegetation. Sunrises are particularly inspiring over the Pequop Mountains to the east.

Camping within the East Humboldt Range is primitive, and around Winchell Lake is no exception. In the absence of developed campsites, make sure you restore your camp area to its original state before leaving. Firewood around the lake is virtually nonexistent, so don't plan on building a campfire unless you're packing firewood. Fishing, however, is reportedly fair for cutthroat trout.

The upper basin provides plenty of opportunities for further exploration, for scrambling up peaks, or for looking for wildlife. In the early evening you may be fortunate enough to be serenaded by coyotes. Although the trail south of the lake is poorly maintained, traveling another 3.5 miles to Lizzie's Basin, in the shadow of 11,306-foot Hole in the Mountain Peak, makes an excellent trip extension.

POSSIBLE ITINERARY

	Camp	Miles	Elevation Gain
Day 1	Winchell Lake	3.0	1010
Day 2	Out	3.0	100

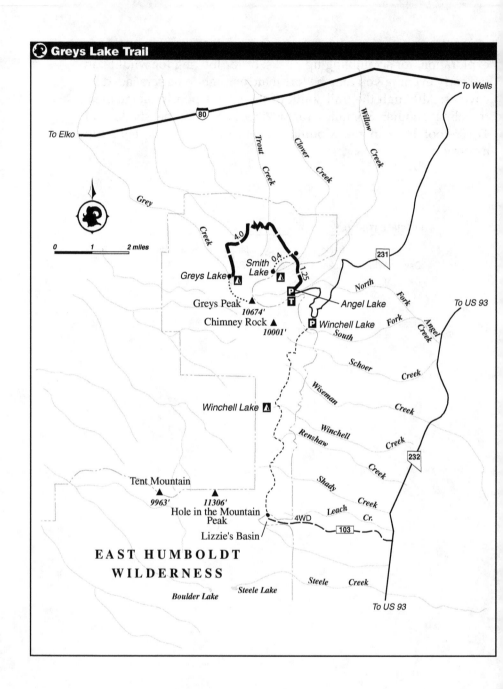

To Wells

To Elko

80

Willow Creek

Trout Creek

Clover Creek

Grey Creek

231

0 1 2 miles

4.0

Smith Lake

0.4

1.25

Greys Lake

North Fork

To US 93

Greys Peak ▲
10674'

Angel Lake

Chimney Rock ▲
10001'

South Fork

Angel Creek

Winchell Lake

Schoer Creek

Wiseman Creek

Winchell Lake ▲

Renshaw

Winchell Creek

232

Creek

Tent Mountain
▲
9963'

▲
11306'
Hole in the Mountain
Peak

Shady Creek

Leach Cr.

4WD

103

Lizzie's Basin

EAST HUMBOLDT
WILDERNESS

Steele Creek

Boulder Lake

Steele Lake

To US 93

9   Greys Lake Trail

RATINGS (1–10)			MILES	ELEVATION GAIN	DAYS	SHUTTLE MILEAGE
Scenery	Solitude	Difficulty				
8	7	6	10.5	3275	2–3	N/A

AREA   East Humboldt Mountains

MAPS   USGS-*Welcome*; USFS-*Ruby Mountains and East Humboldt Wildernesses*

USUALLY OPEN   Early July to mid-October

BEST   Mid-July to mid-August

PERMITS   None

CONTACT   Ruby Mountains Ranger District (775) 752-3357

SPECIAL ATTRACTIONS   Lakes, views, mountain scenery, wildflowers, solitude

PROBLEMS   Infrequently maintained trail, poor campsites

HOW TO GET THERE   From Interstate 80, take the WEST WELLS exit No. 351, turn south onto U.S. 93 and immediately west onto State Route 231, signed ANGEL LAKE. Follow paved road into Forest Service land at 7 miles from the highway, and, 0.3 miles farther, continue past the turnoff to Angel Creek Campground. Soon the road narrows and makes a steep, winding climb up the foothills. At 9.75 miles, in the midst of a hairpin turn, you pass the Winchell Lake trailhead and continue the climb.

    Fine views of Chimney Rock, Greys Peak and a bounty of cascades streaming down the mountainside greet you as you round a curve and continue toward Angel Lake. Before reaching the lake, follow signs for HUMBOLDT NATIONAL FOREST CAMPGROUND and GREYS LAKE TRAIL to the trailhead parking area, where you'll find plenty of

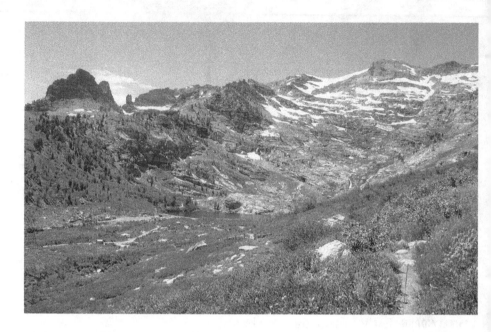

Angel Lake from Greys Lake Trail

parking and restrooms with running water. If you continue all the way to Angel Lake, you will be subject to a day-use fee for parking your car.

INTRODUCTION The Greys Lake Trail leads you from one spectacular subalpine lake to another in five short miles. You may begin your journey amid the hustle and bustle of Angel Lake, where anglers, picnickers, campers, and sightseers mill about, but solitude is quickly gained once you start to make progress up the trail. For much of the summer, you're sure to enjoy not only the wide variety of wildflowers that grace the trail along the way, but the verdant slopes surrounding the lake as well. Once you reach the lake basin, the impressive spires and steep rock walls of the East Humboldt Range present a stirring sight. Wide-ranging views of Starr Valley below with its ranches and circular irrigation patterns are quite pleasing also.

Plenty of options are available for further wanderings for those who don't mind stepping off the trail; an easy cross-country route to remote Smith Lake is within the abilities of most backpackers. More ambitious undertakings could include a climb of Greys Peak or a mountaineer's traverse of the range.

DESCRIPTION Climb away from the upper parking area across a hillside covered with young aspens and wildflowers. About 100 yards from the parking lot, a use-trail from the campground meets the main trail at a switchback. Continue to the top of a short rise, where you reach a steel gate in a fence meant to restrict cattle from overrunning the area around Angel Lake. Gazing back, you have an excellent view of Angel Lake, as Greys Peak and Chimney Rock dominate the skyline above. Continue the climb as the foliage shifts from shrubs and flowers to sagebrush. At the top of a ridge, 0.9 mile from the trailhead, you reach the wilderness boundary.

Beyond the boundary, you follow the trail on a descent toward Clover Creek, passing through dry and rocky terrain. Nearing the creek, lush vegetation begins to flourish again, virtually choking the stream channel with aspens and brush. After crossing the broad but shallow stream, you climb about 75 yards up to a switchback.

Side Trip to Smith Lake: A use-trail branches away from the main trail near the switchback but quickly fades amid the dense brush of the creek bottom. Find the least brushy route up the canyon from this point, which may not be an easy task; you can cross the creek where

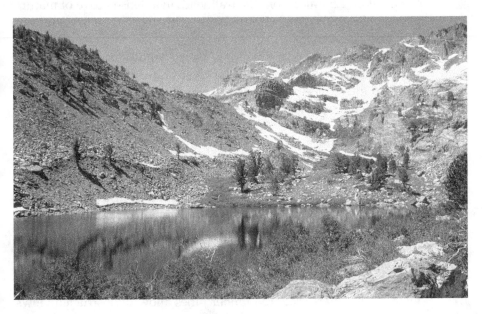

Smith Lake in the East Humboldt Range

the brush is less dense, or find a route away from the creek through the sagebrush. Whichever way you choose, head for a trio of dead snags on the boulder-covered hillside ahead. Eventually the brush lessens, the grade of ascent eases, and you reach the northwest shore of Smith Lake, 0.4 mile from the Greys Lake Trail.

Talus slopes sprinkled with isolated limber pines lead up to the rugged cliffs that rim the clear waters of the lake. Near the outlet, denser stands of limber pine provide a bit of shade for a pair of campsites. Fishing is excellent for cutthroat and golden trout, and American grayling, although, thick brush around the shoreline inhibits access to anglers. A small, human-made dam raises questions about some former purpose. **End of Side Trip**

From the switchback just above Clover Creek, you make a lengthy ascent to the top of another ridge and start a traverse across the northeast slopes of the East Humboldt Range. Views toward the head of the canyon are quite picturesque, with rugged peaks rising above green-carpeted slopes. The traverse takes you to the edge of the broad, sweeping gorge of Trout Creek and the start of a steep, 700-foot descent to the bottom of the canyon. You reach the floor of the canyon, 2.5 miles from the trailhead, in a dense grove of mature aspens. Gingerly cross Trout Creek with the aid of a couple of downed aspen snags.

Beyond the creek, a mile-long, steep, winding ascent leads you out of Trout Creek canyon to the crest of a ridge, passing a well-watered grove of aspens along the way. The long climb ends after a series of switchbacks terminates at a notch below a peak sparsely forested with limber pines, where a large cairn marks the windswept pass.

From the pass, a mild, rocky descent leads to a small, lush meadow, where the trail falters for a short stretch. A well-placed old sign, simply stating TRAIL, points you in the right direction across the meadow. Beyond the meadow, you climb again through limber pines up to the top of yet another ridge, this one just below point 9210 on the USGS map.

From here, a final, one-mile descent is all that stands between you and the lake. The trail switchbacks down from the ridge to a vista point, where scattered limber pines allow unobstructed views of Greys Lake and the surrounding topography. More switchbacks lead you down to the lakeshore, 5.25 miles from Angel Lake.

Greys Lake shimmers in the Great Basin sun, in a canyon rimmed by steep cliffs on the south and west and sloping terrain to the southeast that culminates in the jagged summit of 10,674-foot Greys Peak. These slopes are carpeted with lush grasses and wild-flowers throughout most of the summer, providing a fine comple-ment to the gray rocky cliffs above, where patches of snow cling to the north-facing slopes. Sparkling water rushes down the inlet into the lake from a meadow basin above the south shore. Exiting the lake, the outlet tumbles down the canyon, periodically forming pic-turesque cascades over low rock walls, on the way to join the Humboldt River farther downstream.

Greys Lake offers little in the way of developed campsites. In fact, the entire basin appears pristine, almost untouched. The only truly developed site is above the lake, on the west side near the main trail, a site frequently used by horse packers as a semi-perma-nent base camp, which means backpackers will most likely prefer a less aromatic location. Other possibilities include spots near the out-let, or above the south shore near the inlet. Wherever you decide to camp, firewood is in very short supply. Fishing may be quite good for brook and cutthroat trout, and unlike at Smith Lake, almost the entire shoreline is accessible to anglers.

If further exploration sounds appealing, you can follow a faint use-trail up into the upper basin to find a small pond, a marshy meadow, and even more dramatic views of the cliffs and peaks above. Mountaineers can continue upward to test their skills on a summit attempt of Greys Peak. Although a trail extending beyond Greys Lake running south along the west side of the range is shown on the USGS maps, this trail has not been maintained for years and has disappeared in spots, degenerating into more of a cross-country route than anything close to an actual trail. With the aid of a shuttle, strong parties with good off-trail abilities have traversed the crest of the East Humboldt Mountains on a multi-day outing.

POSSIBLE ITINERARY

	Camp	Miles	Elevation Gain
Day 1	Greys Lake	5.25	1875
Day 2	Out	5.25	1470

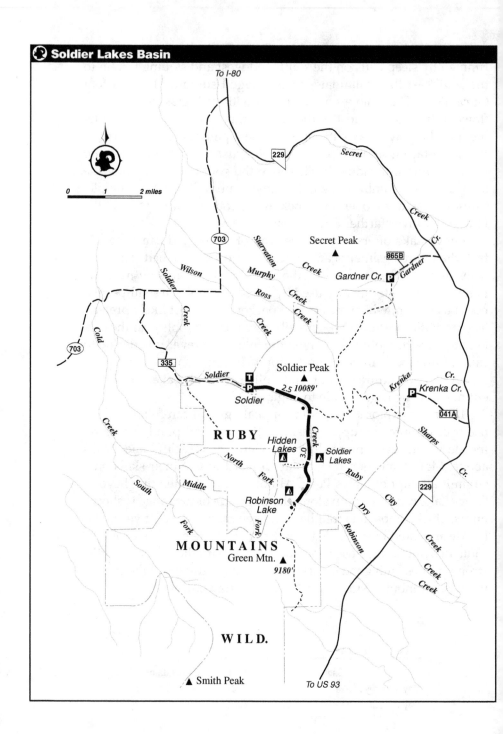

10 Soldier Lakes Basin

RATINGS (1–10)			MILES	ELEVATION GAIN	DAYS	SHUTTLE MILEAGE
Scenery	Solitude	Difficulty				
8	8	6	11	2400	2 – 4	N/A

AREA Ruby Mountains

MAPS USGS-*Soldier Peak, Verdi Peak*; USFS-*Ruby Mountains and East Humboldt Wildernesses*

USUALLY OPEN Mid-June to mid-October

BEST July-August

PERMITS None

CONTACT Humboldt National Forest (775) 738-5171

SPECIAL ATTRACTIONS Lakes, wildflowers, scenery, views

PROBLEMS Cattle

HOW TO GET THERE Take exit No. 321 from Interstate 80, signed HAL-LECK, RUBY VALLEY, and travel on State Route 229 nearly 11 miles to a junction with County Road 703. Following a sign reading LAMOILLE 18, head south on 703, which quickly turns from asphalt to gravel. In 5.3 miles the road bends sharply west, and after another 2 miles you reach a junction, where you should turn onto Soldier Creek Road No. 335. As signs indicate, for the next couple of miles you are passing through private property until reaching the Forest Service boundary—please respect the property rights of the owners. Once you reach government land, the road narrows to a single-lane dirt track with turnouts. Proceed 2.5 miles past the Forest Service boundary to the trailhead at the end of the road, where parking at a grassy flat adjacent to Soldier Creek is available for perhaps a half-dozen cars.

INTRODUCTION Nearly equal to Lamoille Canyon in scenic attributes, the northern section of the Ruby Mountains sees far fewer visitors. Although there are no guarantees that you will be completely alone while traveling in Soldier Lakes Basin, you're more likely to see cows than people. Plenty of lakes, six in all and each with its own charm, provide bountiful opportunities for exploration and enjoyment. The rugged peaks standing guard over the basin will lure explorers and mountaineers as well. If fishing is on your itinerary, this trip is hard to beat as the lakes teem with fish and receive light pressure from anglers. The sunrises are incomparable as well.

The first part of the trail ascends Soldier Creek canyon, holding a boisterous, rowdy stream that tumbles down the narrow gorge amid a diverse collection of wildflowers, shrubs, and trees along the banks. Above the canyon, a broad plateau cradles not only the lakes but a number of wildflower-laden meadows also.

DESCRIPTION Follow the continuation of the old road, boulder-hopping over Soldier Creek and climbing up the north bank, quickly detecting the contrast in vegetation between the roadside, with dry, open hillsides of sagebrush, and the banks of the creek, laden with lush riparian foliage of aspen, mahogany, alder, tobacco brush, and wildflowers—what a difference water makes! Near the beginning of the trail, you have a nice view up the canyon, with green meadows rolling up toward the jagged summit of Soldier Peak. About 100 yards past a gate in a barbed-wire fence, you cross the wilderness boundary. As the canyon narrows, the old roadbed gives way to a steeper, single-track trail, where the creek, never more than a stone's throw away, begins to tumble more precipitously. Rounding a bend, you emerge into the lush foliage of a shady aspen grove.

Continuing up the creek, you reach a side canyon where a mudflow during the winter of 1994-1995 sent tons of debris roaring down the gorge, uprooting trees along the way. After negotiating a path across the debris, you climb moderately steeply on good trail again. Eventually, the canyon widens, the grade moderates, and the more open terrain allows for fine views of Soldier Peak. The path veers away from the creek for a time until you wander back through a field of waist-high wildflowers, crossing a spring-fed tributary along the way. Gradually rising out of Soldier Creek Canyon, you veer south to follow the trail alongside the now tranquil creek, which etches its way through gently rising meadowlands. With a

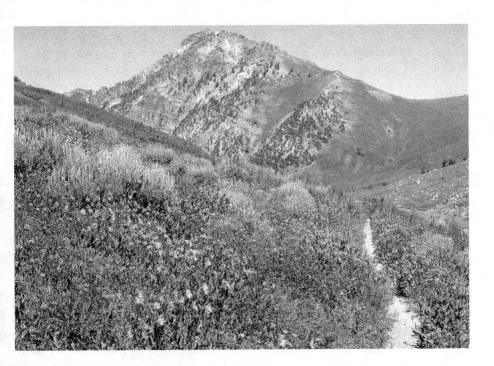

Soldier Peak from the Soldier Lakes Trails

sense of being at the top of the world, you gaze across the broad expanse of a rolling, flower-carpeted basin merging along the fringe with jagged peaks that pierce the azure sky. At 2.5 miles, you come to a signed junction with a faint trail, accessible from the Gardner Creek and Krenka Creek trailheads on the east side of the range.

Following a sign for SOLDIER BASIN, you proceed south on mildly ascending trail, through sagebrush and mixed wildflowers, passing a campsite just off the trail in a small aspen grove. At 3.25 miles, you cross Soldier Creek and continue 0.75 mile through patches of corn lilies to a pair of side streams, the first emanating from a spring 0.5 mile up the hillside, and the second draining Hidden Lakes, a pair of lakes well concealed in a basin near the top of the ridge.

Another 0.5 mile of mild climbing leads past more wildflowers, over the lip of Soldier Basin to the first Soldier Lake, a small, oblong, shallow pond surrounded by sagebrush and flowers, with a row of aspens and pines along the far shore. About 100 yards downhill is a second, slightly larger lake, near the headwaters of Soldier Creek. Campsites are very limited at both lakes, but seem sufficient for the few backpackers who stay overnight.

Warning: Cattle grazing is the major drawback to camping in the Soldier Lakes Basin. Even if you're fortunate enough to evade these "wild" beasts, you probably won't be able to avoid their excrement, so choose your water source wisely, and don't forget your filter!

Away from the first two lakes, you ascend a short rise and contour around to the crossing of the creek draining the largest of the Soldier Lakes, where you'll find that plenty of potential campsites abound, scattered amid the low-growing shrubs around the lake. Just over a low rise to the east you'll discover three small ponds. According to the Forest Service, brook trout reside in all the Soldier Lakes.

Side Trip to Hidden Lakes: Although the USGS map shows a trail from Soldier Lakes to Hidden Lake, the lower part has virtually disappeared. From the outlet of the largest Soldier Lake, climb northwest from the trail up a sagebrush-covered ridge for about 0.5 mile to a prominent white rock perched on a knoll. Near the rock you can follow a faint path on a nearly level traverse south into the canyon of the outlet. Make a short drop into this narrow gorge and head upstream toward the lakes, climbing steeply at times. Periodic cairns may help to guide you, but the route is straightforward.

Hidden Lakes, although two bodies of water, appear to be more of a single lake separated by a thin, grass-covered isthmus holding a row of limber pines. The lakes sit in a narrow bowl, almost at the crest of the range. A stand of limber pine graces the southwest shore and runs up toward the summit of Peak 9963. Views are excellent of the basin below and the East Humboldt Mountains to the northeast. The sunrises from this lofty perch are awe-inspiring. A use-trail leads up to the top of a minor ridge at the north end of the lake, offering even better views, as well as a campsite near a character-rich limber-pine snag. Other campsites, within easier reach of water, can be found on the east shore. A healthy population of cutthroat trout will test the skill of anglers. **End of Side Trip**

Wander away from the largest Soldier Lake, on a level course before a mild descent takes you past small ponds toward Robinson Lake. Near the bottom of the descent, the trail divides; the main path branches left and proceeds to the lake near the outlet. The right-hand path heads across a spring-fed channel of Robinson Creek to the east shore.

Robinson is easily the largest of the lakes in the northern Rubies, and certainly one of the most scenic, cradled below towering cliffs. Green, sloping hillsides merge with gray slabs of angled rock beneath jagged summits of peaks over 10,000 feet high, dramatically reflected in the sky-blue water. Brook trout are so numerous that anglers may start to hallucinate about being able to walk across their backs from one side to the other.

Warning: Although a path encircles the lake, the north end is so concentrated with springs that passage over the saturated soil is difficult and ecologically damaging.

A spring-fed cascade flows down vertical cliffs on the west shore, providing a reliable place to filter water. Backpackers will find limited campsites near the outlet and at the end of the trail on the east side of the lake.

Tip: Bring a dependable stove, as firewood is virtually nonexistent.

Potential for further exploration of the northern Rubies abounds, including heading south along the continuation of the deteriorating trail into Withington Basin, a verdant, sloping vale fed by numerous streams, beneath meadow-clad, aptly-named Green Mountain. The short climb up the saddle between Withington and Soldier Lakes basins is well worth the effort for the views alone. Cross-country enthusiasts can explore the crest of the range above Soldier Lakes Basin without too much difficulty.

POSSIBLE ITINERARY

	Camp	Miles	Elevation Gain
Day 1	Robinson Lake	5.5	2400
Day 2	Out	5.5	100

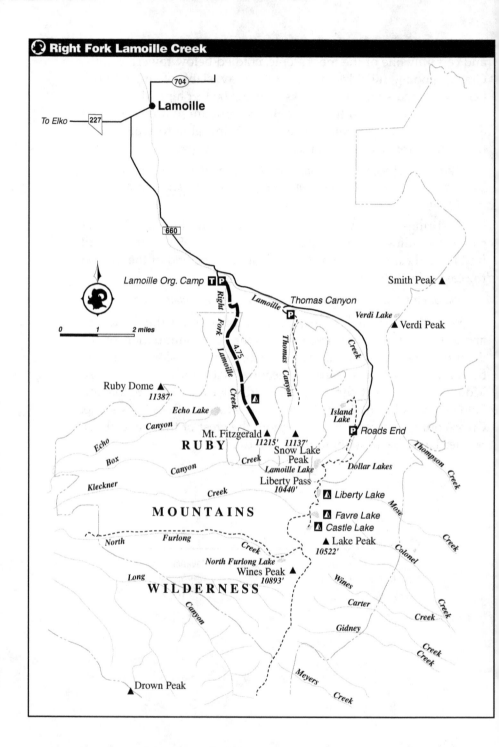

Lamoille

704

To Elko — 227

660

Lamoille Org. Camp

Smith Peak ▲

Right Fork

Lamoille

Thomas Canyon

Verdi Lake

Verdi Peak ▲

0 1 2 miles

4.75

Lamoille Creek

Thomas Canyon

Creek

Ruby Dome ▲
11387'

Echo Lake

Island
Lake

Canyon

Mt. Fitzgerald ▲
11215'

▲
11137'

Roads End

RUBY

Snow Lake
Peak

Echo

Box

Creek

Lamoille Lake

Dollar Lakes

Canyon

Liberty Pass
10440'

Kleckner

Creek

Liberty Lake

MOUNTAINS

Favre Lake

Castle Lake

North

Furlong

Creek

▲ Lake Peak
10522'

Colonel

Creek

North Furlong Lake

Long

Wines Peak ▲
10893'

Wines

WILDERNESS

Carter

Creek

Canyon

Gidney

Creek
Creek

Meyers

Drown Peak ▲

Creek

Thompson Creek

Mose

11 Right Fork Lamoille Creek

RATINGS (1–10)			MILES	ELEVATION GAIN	DAYS	SHUTTLE MILEAGE
Scenery	Solitude	Difficulty				
9	9	7	9.5	2700	2–3	N/A

AREA Ruby Mountains

MAPS USGS-*Lamoille*; USFS-*Ruby Mountains and East Humboldt Wildernesses*

USUALLY OPEN Late June to mid-October

BEST July-August

PERMITS None

CONTACT Humboldt National Forest (775) 738-5171

SPECIAL ATTRACTIONS Outstanding mountain scenery, wildflowers, solitude

PROBLEMS Sections of poor trail

HOW TO GET THERE From Interstate 80 take exit No. 301 signed ELKO DOWNTOWN and head south for 0.8 mile to a left-hand turn onto Business 80. Proceed another 0.8 mile to 5th Street and turn right onto State Route 228, following signs for SPRING CREEK, LAMOILLE and JIGGS. Drive out of old downtown Elko, cross the railroad tracks and the Humboldt River on an overpass, and turn left at a traffic signal, still on S.R. 228. You quickly pass the Humboldt National Forest ranger station on the left at Last Chance Road, and continue on four-lane highway, cresting Lamoille Summit at 5.5 miles from I-80, where you have a fine view of the Ruby Mountains in the distance.

Two miles from Lamoille Summit, S.R. 228 intersects S.R. 227, and you proceed straight, now on S.R. 227. About 5 miles past the

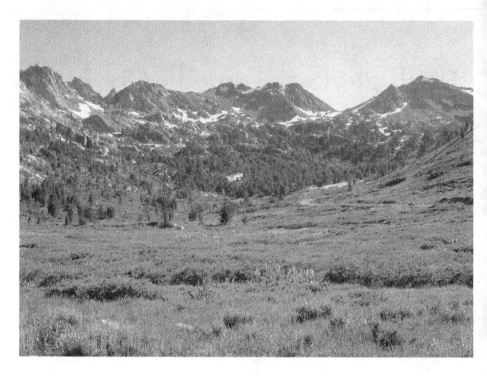

Lamoille Canyon

intersection, the road narrows to two lanes and you continue toward the small community of Lamoille.

About 0.5 mile before you reach Lamoille, 7.5 miles from the intersection between 227 and 228, turn right onto Forest Road 660, also designated Lamoille Canyon Scenic Highway, following a sign marked LAMOILLE CANYON RECREATION AREA. After 2.5 miles, you enter Forest Service land, pass Powerhouse Picnic Area and proceed into glacier-carved Lamoille Canyon. Continue up the canyon to the turnoff for Camp Lamoille, 5 miles from the junction with S.R. 227, and follow the gravel road to the wide parking area on the right, just before the gate into Camp Lamoille.

INTRODUCTION Only 2 miles from a popular summer camp lies a seldom visited, flourishing valley rimmed by steep canyon walls and towering peaks, a hidden jewel that is one of the Ruby Mountains most priceless treasures. The trail passes through some of the most luxuriant vegetation you'll find anywhere in Nevada, alongside one of the most rambunctious creeks, and into a dramatic hanging valley of glacial origin that any mountain range would welcome. Boundless alpine scenery and opportunities for off-trail exploration await the visitor who is willing to invest a bit of effort to reach this truly spectacular area. Despite the unparalleled beauty, the upper canyon of the Right Fork Lamoille Creek is not afforded wilderness protection (a concession to a local heli-skiing operation), but the area is as pristine and magnificent as any in the Ruby Mountains.

DESCRIPTION From the parking area, continue up the road through Camp Lamoille to the edge of the development, near some A-frame cabins. Follow a twin-tracked jeep road that eventually reverts to single-track trail and walk through young aspens toward the creek. Nearing the creek, the path turns upstream to a fork, where you follow the right-hand branch upstream for a short distance to another informal junction. Follow the main trail to the left to a ford of the creek (the right-hand path heads upstream to a dramatic series of short cascades which tumble over rock cliffs).

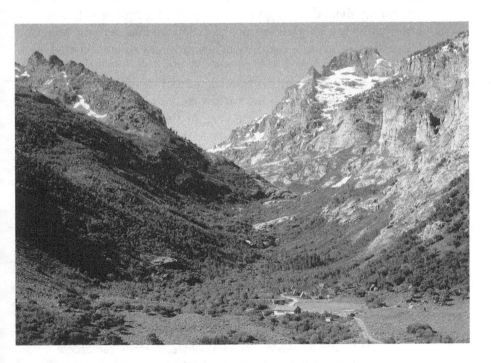

The canyon of Right Fork Lamoille Creek

Mt. Fitzgerald

Mt. Fitzgerald (11,215') is one of the most alpine-looking peaks in the Ruby Mountains. Unlike most geographic appellations in Nevada, the name of the mountain came fairly recently, to honor John Fitzgerald Kennedy, 35th president of the United States.

Ford the creek and follow the trail on the east side of the creek through grasses, shrubs, and wildflowers, including monkey flower, columbine, and lupine. Soon the trail forsakes the bottom of the valley and begins a steep, switchbacking climb amid dense stands of aspen and lush trailside vegetation. At the top of the switchbacks, the grade eases and you make a long, gentle ascent, still through lush foliage. At 1.5 miles, you pass into the Ruby Mountains Wilderness and eventually start climbing more steeply.

The vegetation temporarily opens up enough to reveal a series of ponds below the trail, until thick brush and tall aspens return, providing shaded passage across a pair of gurgling side streams. Eventually, the jungle-like foliage is left behind, as you ascend a succession of granite slabs, benches, and clearings accented by a brilliant display of wildflowers. Follow a deteriorating path through aspens and brush to an apparent dead-end at a massive rock wall that pinches off the narrow canyon. Tenuously clinging to a very slim path between the base of the rock and the churning creek, you circumvent this obstacle to find distinct trail again. Heading away from the raucous creek, the ascent leads across more cliffs and slabs to the lip of the upper basin.

Heading into the magnificent hanging valley of the upper canyon, the tread diminishes in the lush vegetation near a beaver pond, but despite the lack of a bona fide trail, the wide-open nature of the area makes for straightforward navigation. The basin is a verdant, glacier-carved vale bisected by a clear stream coursing below serrated ridges and rugged peaks. Although developed campsites are virtually nonexistent, plenty of potential sites will easily accommodate backpackers. Mountaineers should find abundant pitches and peaks to satiate their appetites, including Mt. Fitzgerald.

Tip: Hardy and experienced cross-country enthusiasts can accept the challenge of a rugged route over the crest and across the slopes above Box Canyon to isolated Echo Lake.

	Camp	Miles	Elevation Gain
Day 1	Right Fork Lamoille Creek	4.75	2600
Day 2	Out	4.75	100

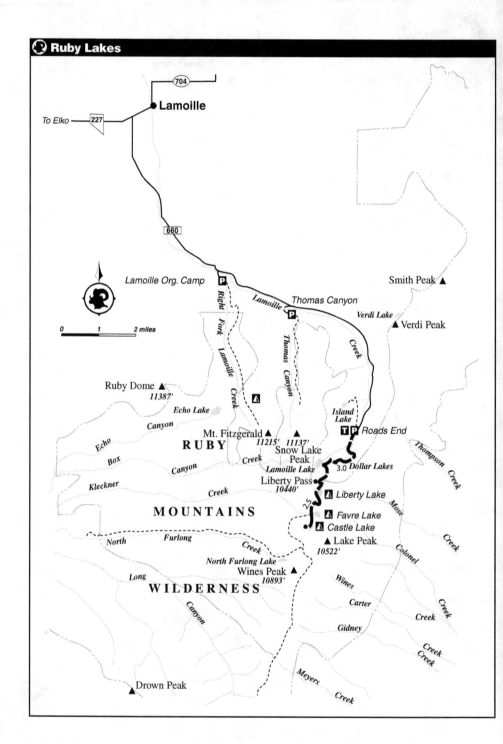

704

To Elko — 227

● Lamoille

660

Lamoille Org. Camp

Right Fork Lamoille Creek

Lamoille

Thomas Canyon

Thomas Canyon

Smith Peak ▲

Verdi Lake

▲ Verdi Peak

Creek

0   1   2 miles

Ruby Dome ▲
11387'

Echo Lake

Canyon

Echo Box

Kleckner

Mt. Fitzgerald ▲
11215' 11137' ▲

RUBY

Creek

Canyon

Creek

Island Lake

T P Roads End

Snow Lake Peak

Lamoille Lake

3.0 Dollar Lakes

Thompson Creek

MOUNTAINS

North Furlong

Creek

North Furlong Lake

Long

Canyon

WILDERNESS

Liberty Pass
10440'

2.5

▲ Liberty Lake

Mose Creek

▲ Favre Lake

▲ Castle Lake

▲ Lake Peak
10522'

Colonel Creek

Wines Peak ▲
10893'

Wines

Carter Creek

Gidney

Creek Creek

Drown Peak ▲

Meyers Creek

12 Ruby Lakes

RATINGS (1–10)			MILES	ELEVATION GAIN	DAYS	SHUTTLE MILEAGE
Scenery	Solitude	Difficulty				
10	7	7	11	2950	2–4	N/A

AREA Ruby Mountains

MAPS USGS-*Ruby Dome*; USFS-*Ruby Mountains and East Humboldt Wildernesses*

USUALLY OPEN Mid-July to mid-October

BEST Mid-July to August

PERMITS None

CONTACT Humboldt National Forest (775) 738-5171

SPECIAL ATTRACTIONS Lakes, wildflowers, scenery, views

PROBLEMS High altitude, possibile snow-covered trail below pass

HOW TO GET THERE From Interstate 80 take exit No. 301 signed ELKO DOWNTOWN and head south for 0.8 mile to a left-hand turn onto Business 80. Proceed another 0.8 mile to 5th Street and turn right onto State Route 228, following signs for SPRING CREEK, LAMOILLE and JIGGS. Drive out of old downtown Elko, cross the railroad tracks and the Humboldt River on an overpass, and turn left at a traffic signal, still on S.R. 228. You quickly pass the Humboldt National Forest ranger station on the left at Last Chance Road, and continue on four-lane highway, cresting Lamoille Summit at 5.5 miles from I-80, where you have a fine view of the Ruby Mountains in the distance.

Two miles from Lamoille Summit, S.R. 228 intersects S.R. 227, and you proceed straight ahead, now on S.R. 227. About 5 miles past the intersection, the road narrows to two lanes and you continue toward the small community of Lamoille.

About 0.5 mile before you reach Lamoille, 7.5 miles from the intersection between 227 and 228, turn right onto Forest Road 660, also designated Lamoille Canyon Scenic Highway, following a sign marked LAMOILLE CANYON RECREATION AREA. After 2.5 miles, you enter Forest Service land, pass Powerhouse Picnic Area and proceed into glacier-carved Lamoille Canyon. Continue up the Lamoille Canyon Scenic Highway to the parking area in the turnaround at the end of the road, 12.5 miles from State Route 227, where you'll find pit toilets, running water, picnic tables, and horse loading facilities.

INTRODUCTION The climb over Liberty Pass and into the Ruby Lakes is the most popular backpack in the Ruby Mountains. If you ask backpackers whether they have ever been to the Rubies and the answer is yes, then invariably this is the trail they hiked—and with good reason. In a relatively few miles (unfortunately the elevation gain is not small) hikers can enter the subalpine, glacier-carved basin at the head of Kleckner Creek canyon, where three cirque-bound lakes repose below rugged, pinnacled ridges. Most hikers are content just to reach magnificent Liberty Lake on the far side of 10,440-foot Liberty Pass, but Favre and Castle lakes are worth the extra effort, providing opportunities for increased solitude. On the trailhead side of the pass are the Dollar Lakes, a pair of symmetrical lakelets surrounded by green meadow and, in stark contrast, austere Lamoille Lake, where nearly barren slopes create an alpine appearance. Toss in delightful Lamoille Creek, spectacular wildflower displays, great views, and excellent fishing opportunities and you have all the ingredients for a classic backcountry experience.

DESCRIPTION Begin the climb toward Liberty Pass on a moderate grade through open terrain bordering rushing Lamoille Creek. A bevy of trailside wildflowers greets you, including corn lily, larkspur, lupine, paintbrush, and yarrow. The downstream views of Lamoille Canyon become more impressive with the gain in elevation. One-third mile from the trailhead, you cross the creek on a wooden bridge and continue up the east bank, where pines start to appear. At 0.6 mile the trail bends sharply east and crosses the branch of creek that drains the Dollar Lakes. After two more stream crossings, you skirt the north edge of the lakes. A steep ridge above the far shore adds a rugged backdrop to the pristine ponds, which are bordered by grassy meadows and lush willows. Anglers should keep going, as the shallow lakes are reportedly devoid of fish.

A gentle, 0.2-mile climb leads away from Dollar Lakes to much larger Lamoille Lake, cradled in a deep gouge near the west edge of the upper canyon. The steep walls at the head of the canyon rising up towards Liberty Pass make the lake seem rugged and forbidding. The treeless shore appears almost lifeless, but willow brush and grasses thrive in the alpine-like environment. A few campsites are scattered around the north shore, but most visitors seem content with just a brief visit—hikers enjoy a picnic lunch, and anglers ply the waters for brook trout.

Once past the placid waters of Lamoille Lake, the trail becomes increasingly steep for the duration of the 700-foot climb through rocky terrain to the pass. The type of lush vegetation along the first part of the trail is not found above the lake—eventually even the hardy limber pines grudgingly give in to the harsh conditions. Near the pass, ice and snow cling to the crevices in north-facing walls well into summer.

Warning: *Patches of snow will most likely be found on parts of the trail below the pass in early season, and may even cover the path entirely after a winter of heavy snowfall Check with the Forest Service for current conditions before your trip.*

After 3 miles and 1600 feet, you stand atop Liberty Pass, where the view is excellent; spend enough time to soak in the incredible vista, as well as to catch your breath before rushing off to the lakes below. South along the crest, Lake Peak and Wines Peak grab the eye.

At the pass, you cross into Ruby Mountains Wilderness and begin the steep descent toward Liberty Lake, which remains hidden from sight, tucked back well into the head of the canyon. Suddenly, the lake pops into view, creating a dramatic mountain scene, as the deep-blue waters reflect vertical cliffs of dark metamorphic rock. The trail passes well above the west shore of the lake before reaching a lateral, 0.5 mile from the pass. This short path leads to the south shore of the lake near the outlet.

Liberty is the quintessential mountain lake, with splendid scenery and excellent views. Seeing it cradled in a steep-walled

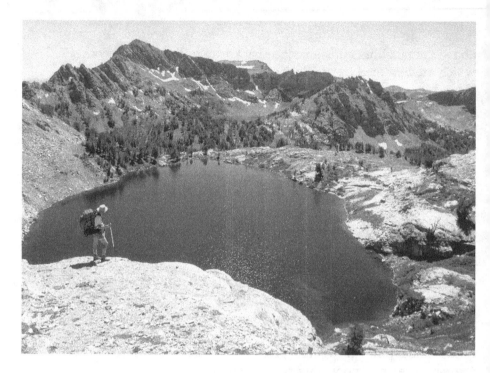

Hiker overlooking Liberty Lake in the Ruby Mountains

basin of rock, perched high above the surrounding canyon, you can appreciate the popularity of this lake. Ironically, travelers along Interstate 80, a mere 30 air miles away, race past the range completely unaware of this tremendous beauty, assuming Nevada is nothing more than endless sagebrush and brown-tinged mountains.

Campsites are plentiful here but firewood is not—be sure to bring a stove if you anticipate hot food or drink. Fishing is good for brook trout.

Warning: *The fragile ecosystem around the lake requires that you observe minimum-impact techniques while camping.*

To visit Favre Lake, return to the Ruby Crest Trail and proceed down the north side of the canyon for 1.25 miles to a use-trail heading east. Follow this path a short distance past a campsite beneath a lone limber pine to the outlet near the west shore, where a wonderful swath of wildflower-covered meadow lines the banks. Cross the creek with the aid of rocks and logs to some campsites amid low pines. Favre Lake, at 9500 feet, sits in a broad, open bowl at the head of Kleckner Creek canyon, surrounded by green, sloping hillsides

Castle and Favre Lakes

Don't look too long at the rugged cliffs of Lake Peak above Castle Lake searching for the lake's namesake — there is no castle. Both Castle and Favre lakes were named after Forest Service employees, Saxon Castle and Clarence Favre.

that gently dip toward the lake. The rugged, gray cliffs along the north ridge of Lake Peak highlight the limber-pine-carpeted hillside above the southeast shore. Pockets of willow may prevent anglers from capturing the brook trout inhabiting the lake, although access is good on the east side. Despite the fine stand of limber pine shading pleasant campsites along the south shore, firewood is scarce.

Although a defined trail up to Castle Lake is nonexistent, the route is straightforward and only 0.25-mile long. A use-trail from the south shore of Favre Lake climbs the steep hillside up to the lip of the basin, where the grade mellows considerably. Another 0.1 mile of easy hiking leads to the north shore.

Castle Lake is a delightful place to spend a couple of hours or a couple of days. Carved out of a steep, horseshoe-shaped basin and flanked by the precipitous cliffs of Lake Peak, Castle Lake has more of an alpine flavor than pastoral Favre Lake. Patches of snow cling to crevices in the gray rock walls of Lake Peak well into summer, adding to the alpine atmosphere. The shoreline is embraced by meadows dotted with willows, with occasional stands of limber pine inching their way up the lower slopes of the basin. Backpackers will find campsites at the north end near the outlet. Unlike at Favre, firewood should be in good supply.

Tip: Don't unpack your fishing pole, as according to the Forest Service, there are no fish in Castle lake. However, the little bit of effort involved in reaching Castle Lake should reap extra dividends in solitude.

POSSIBLE ITINERARY

	Camp	Miles	Elevation Gain
Day 1	Castle Lake	5.5	1950
Day 2	Out	5.5	1000

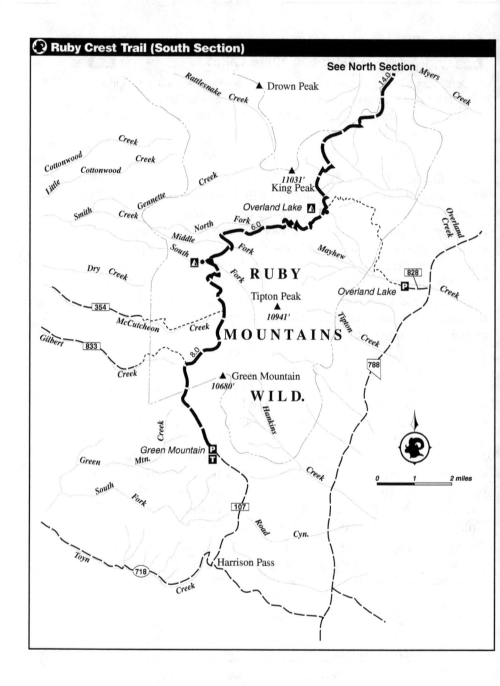

13 Ruby Crest Trail

RATINGS (1–10)			MILES	ELEVATION GAIN	DAYS	SHUTTLE MILEAGE
Scenery	Solitude	Difficulty				
10	10	7	34	9700	3–5	57

AREA Ruby Mountains

MAPS USGS-*Harrison Pass, Franklin Lake SW, Green Mountain, Franklin Lake NW, Ruby Dome*; USFS-*Ruby Mountains and East Humboldt Wildernesses*

USUALLY OPEN Mid-July to mid-October

BEST Mid-July to August

PERMITS None

CONTACT Humboldt National Forest (775) 738-5171

SPECIAL ATTRACTIONS Lakes, wildflowers, scenery, views

PROBLEMS 10-mile stretch without water, high altitude, possibility of snow-covered trail below pass

HOW TO GET THERE *START:* Follow State Route 228 southbound, paralleling the west side of the Ruby Mountains, to the small town of Jiggs, about 27 miles south of the junction with State Route 227. About 3.5 miles beyond Jiggs, the road inauspiciously becomes County Road 718, and turns to gravel 3 miles farther on. Just beyond the Zaga Ranch the road bends and climbs to the east, reaching Harrison Pass, approximately 17 miles from Jiggs.

From the pass, your progress up Forest Road 107 will depend upon the type of vehicle you're driving. Sedans should either park in a large, grassy field near the pass, or drive gingerly up the road 0.5 mile to a pull-out just large enough for a horse trailer. High-clearance vehicles can proceed along the narrow dirt track to a gate

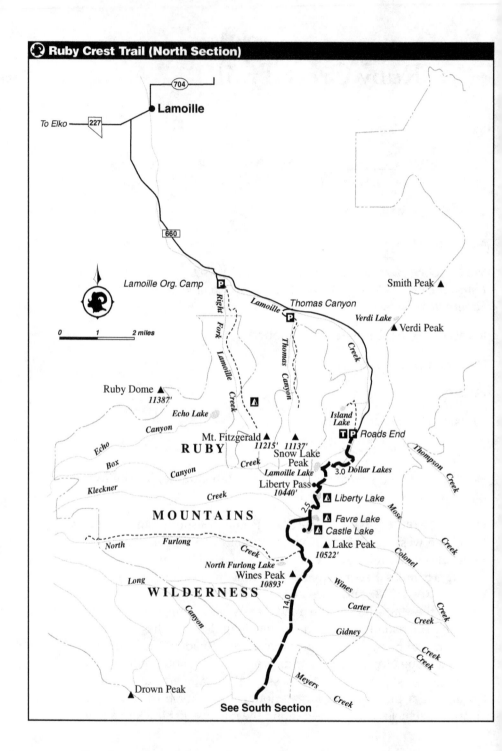

704

Lamoille

To Elko — 227

660

Lamoille Org. Camp [P]

Smith Peak ▲

Right Fork Lamoille Creek

Lamoille

Thomas Canyon [P]

Thomas Canyon

Lamoille Creek

Verdi Lake

▲ Verdi Peak

Thomas Canyon

0   1   2 miles

Ruby Dome ▲
11387'

Echo Lake

Canyon

Echo

Box

Kleckner

[▲]

Mt. Fitzgerald ▲
RUBY   11215' 11137'
            Snow Lake
Creek   Peak
        Lamoille Lake
Canyon   Liberty Pass
            10440'

Island
Lake

[T][P] Roads End

Creek

3.0 Dollar Lakes

2.5

[▲] Liberty Lake

Thompson Creek

Creek

MOUNTAINS

[▲] Favre Lake
[▲] Castle Lake

Mose

North   Furlong
            Creek
        North Furlong Lake
WILDERNESS Wines Peak ▲
                10893'

Long

Canyon

▲ Lake Peak
    10522'

Colonel

Creek

14.0

Wines

Carter

Creek

Gidney

Creek

Creek

Creek

Drown Peak ▲

Meyers   Creek

See South Section

at 0.9 mile. Just past the gate is the roughest and steepest section, where some drivers may elect to activate the four-wheel-drive. Beyond this obstacle, the road parallels a fence and then bends northwest. Approximately 100 yards before a large rock outcrop that towers over a stand of aspens, you reach a sign reading VEHICLE TRAFFIC NOT ADVISED BEYOND THIS POINT, and find parking nearby in a grassy area. Travel beyond the sign is not particularly difficult, but parking spaces are virtually nonexistent.

END: Follow the description in Trip 12 (p. 131) to the parking area in the turnaround at the end of the road, 12.5 miles from State Route 227, where you'll find pit toilets, running water, picnic tables and horse-loading facilities.

INTRODUCTION Considered by many the preeminent trail in Nevada, the Ruby Crest National Recreation Trail offers backpackers and equestrians one of the best wilderness experiences in the state. Mountain lakes, absent from the majority of the rest of Nevada's backcountry, are here in abundance, including Overland, North Furlong, Favre, Castle, Liberty, Lamoille, and the two Dollar Lakes. Even more unusual is a spectacular waterfall, found in the Overland Creek basin.

Superb views are nearly constant companions, and a scenic calendar could easily be compiled from the photo opportunities along this trail. In addition, during peak season, the Ruby Mountains offer one of the best wildflower displays anywhere in the state, as well as many pristine meadows. Wildlife enthusiasts will enjoy searching for mountain goats, Rocky Mountain bighorn sheep, mule deer, and a wide variety of fowl, including raptors such as golden eagles and red-tailed hawks. Even the fishing can be fantastic.

The few descriptions of the Ruby Crest Trail in print start in Lamoille Canyon and end at the Green Mountain trailhead near Harrison Pass. This description reverses that direction, advocating a journey from south to north for excellent reasons. Since most recreationists will view the Ruby Lakes as the highlight of the route, traveling south to north saves the climax for the end. In addition, most backpackers will appreciate the descent from Liberty Pass rather than the steep climb up from Lamoille Canyon. Another benefit of hiking in this direction is having the intense summer sun on your back rather than in your eyes. Feel free to select your own

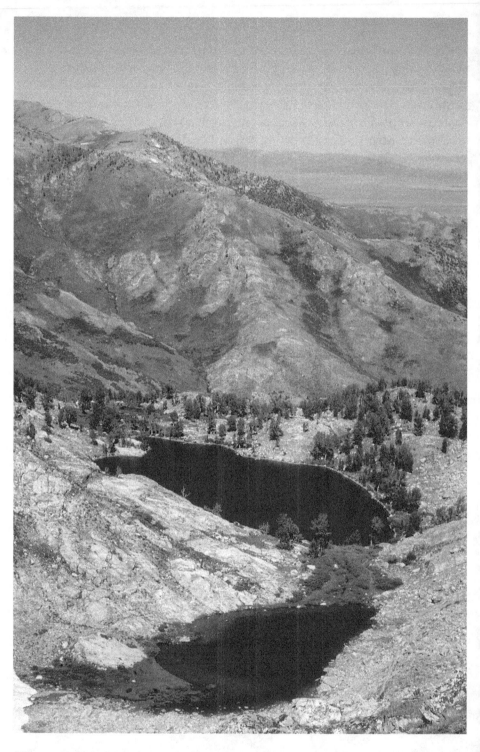

Tarn and Overland Lake from Ruby Crest

direction, but traveling from south to north is preferable for the average backpacker.

Warning: *Although this trip can be idyllic, there are a few cautions worth noting. First, Liberty Pass, at the north end of the trail, is high (10,400'±), with a north-facing slope that may harbor high-angled snowfields well into summer. Make sure you're acclimated and, in the early part of the season, prior to your arrival at the trailhead be sure to check with the Forest Service about current conditions, as you might need crampons and an ice axe. Second, there is no water in the 10-mile middle section of the route, so carry extra water between the last branch of Overland Creek and the springs above North Furlong Creek. Last, the one-way trip requires a lengthy car shuttle—make sure you allow enough time for the journey between trailheads and make sure your vehicle has enough gas.*

DESCRIPTION Continue up the twin-tracked jeep road, where views to the west over sagebrush-covered slopes are expansive, interrupted only by sporadic stands of aspen. After you pass a large rock outcrop, the grade increases and the tread becomes rocky. Continue along the road to a trail junction in a saddle where a sign reads RUBY CREST TRAIL (ahead) and GREEN MOUNTAIN CREEK (left).

Warning: *Although several trails intersect the southern part of the Ruby Crest Trail, these trails eventually enter private land and there is no public access across to the west.*

At the junction the road gives way to single-track trail, on which you descend about 200 yards to the Ruby Mountains Wilderness boundary before continuing on a descending traverse around the slopes of Green Mountain. Aside from the stream canyons and spring-fed slopes that harbor riparian foliage, most of the terrain along the south end of the Ruby Crest Trail is open grasslands sprinkled with scattered wildflowers. As you continue along the path, a series of interesting rock domes springs into view in the canyon below.

The arid vegetation eventually gives way to a lush display of wildflowers and young aspens as you continue the descending traverse around Green Mountain, aptly-named for the green carpet of shrubs covering its flanks. In a grove of aspens, you reach a three-way junction with Trail No. 050, signed HARRISON LAMOILLE TRAIL, 0.75 mile past the wilderness boundary.

You climb to a shady grove of tall aspens and lush wildflowers, where a nearby spring trickles across the trail and into a beaver pond. Quickly hop across another small stream and curve around the north ridge of Green Mountain to the crossing of McCutcheon Creek, 1 mile from the last junction. Immediately after the crossing, you encounter a junction with Trail No. 049.

From the junction, you follow a mildly ascending traverse before a short, steep climb leads to a saddle in the ridge separating the McCutcheon Creek and Smith Creek watersheds. A series of long-legged switchbacks drops you almost 1500 feet in nearly 2 miles, on the way to South Fork Smith Creek. Although you may not find any developed campsites, plenty of potential exists beneath the shelter of aspens lining this rushing stream. To complete the setting, you have a fine view up the canyon of green hillsides rising up to dramatic rock cliffs, although grazing cattle and their byproducts may be a drawback. Unless you're in a hurry to complete the trip, at nearly 8 miles from the trailhead, this would be a fine place to spend the first night.

From the creek, you quickly ascend the dry hillside to a knob along the crest, and then follow a lengthier descent across the lush, north-facing hillside of the narrow Middle Fork. At the bottom of the steep canyon, you hop across the cramped creek and climb up the steep far bank. Due to the steep nature of the topography, don't expect to find any places to camp along the Middle Fork.

A stiff climb takes you to the top of the ridge and excellent views of the ranges to the west. Unlike in the previous two canyons, the trail doesn't drop to the creek but instead makes a mild ascent across the south wall toward the head of the North Fork's canyon. Small aspens and an abundant display of wildflowers grace the path as you head up the drainage. As you climb gently east, the goal of the next section of trail looms at the ridgecrest, 2.5 miles away and 2000 feet above. A short descent takes you to a Y-junction with Smith Creek Trail No. 109, which descends 0.2 mile to a crossing of North Fork Smith Creek and then heads downstream along the north bank, where you can find adequate campsites.

Away from the junction, the trail begins a more serious ascent, emerging into open slopes of sagebrush, grasses, and wildflowers. You cross a dry drainage and, about 50 feet farther, a willow-lined creeklet, the last water before the Overland Lake basin. On the far bank, a use-trail descends the drainage to connect to the Smith Creek Trail.

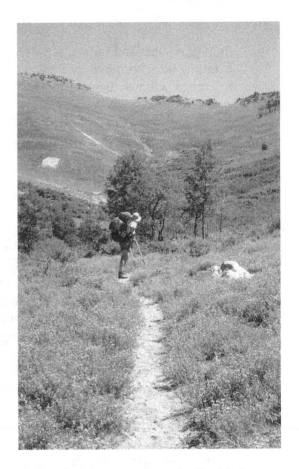

Backpacker below pass above Overland Lake

The trail becomes even steeper beyond the creeklet, as you follow a series of switchbacks that will continue until you've conquered the pass above Overland Lake. Such a long uphill grind is usually the time for repetitive, mind-numbing songs to play in your head, or for deep, meaningful questions like, "Why am I doing this?" An appropriate question for this particular circumstance is, "Why do they call this the Ruby Crest Trail?" Good question, since the last time you were anywhere near the crest of the range was in the car on the approach to the trailhead. Eventually, above the Overland Lake basin, you'll actually be astride the spine of the Rubies for quite a while. In the meantime, you continue the long, dry ascent through sagebrush and grasses, finally reaching the crest near a rock outcrop, 13 miles from the trailhead. An old sign, letters worn away by the harsh elements, testifies to the extreme conditions at the apex of the range. Views of Ruby Valley, Franklin Lakes, and the Pequop Mountains open up to the east. Rather than immediately descending toward Overland Lake, the trail scrambles along the ridge to a rocky viewpoint, where the previously hidden lake and the small tarn above it instantly spring into view.

Switchbacks wind through the barren, rocky terrain of the upper basin, down to the oblong tarn just above the lake, where light-gray cliffs and talus rim the shore. A clear, cold stream gushes from the tarn, bordered by a thin strip of verdant meadow above a thicket of willows. Beyond the willows, the outlet plunges steeply over rocky slopes to the lake below. For a moment, forgetting that you're in Nevada is quite easy, as the alpine scenery seems more reminiscent of the High Sierra or the Rocky Mountains.

You descend through waist-high willows alongside the outlet before the trail moves away from the stream to zigzag across a flower-strewn meadow filled with buttercup, aster, paintbrush, lupine, and shooting star. Contour above the east shore past a camp-site sheltered by limber pines and drop down to the far end of Overland Lake near an old cabin, 14 miles from the trailhead.

Overland Lake is an oval body of clear, green-tinged water occupying a rugged bowl just below the crest of the range, where talus slopes and rock slabs rise up to steep gray and tan peaks rimming the basin on three sides. Limber pines gracefully add a dose of character to the shoreline. Swimming in the chilly waters will be refreshing on a hot summer day, and fishing for brook trout should be good. Although lightly used, Overland Lake is a common stop for parties hiking the Ruby Crest Trail, and for weekenders on the 6-mile Overland Lake Trail (see Trip 14, p. 155).

A few campsites are available near the cabin, but the best site is west of the outlet beneath some tall pines. Most equestrians tether their horses on the east side of the creek and set up camp a good distance downstream—hopefully this practice will continue. Firewood is extremely scarce.

The Ruby Crest Trail heads downhill from the vicinity of the cabin, initially through a patch of alders and wildflowers, then through a boulder field dotted with scattered pines. After 0.4 mile, you intersect the Overland Lake Trail coming up from Ruby Valley below.

The next 4 miles of trail traverse the expansive Overland Creek basin, where excellent mountain scenery offers green hillsides, clear and cold streams, and towering grayish-rock peaks. From the junction, you descend, steeply at times, occasionally switchbacking through meadows filled with wildflowers and scattered limber pines, and eventually reach the first of the many tributaries of Overland Creek, cascading picturesquely down rock slabs. The path heads below the slabs and begins the long traverse of the canyon.

Overland Lake

Unlike many other geographical features in the Rubies, this lake wasn't named for a local settler, but for the Overland Farm, which supplied feed to the horses of the Overland Mail Company, which served the residents of Ruby Valley during the 1860s. Clarence King, famed surveyor, explorer, and mountaineer of the Sierra, named the lake Marian for his sister, but the name was short lived. The old cabin at the north end of the lake looks old enough to have some history as well, but is of fairly recent origin, used by modern-day horse packers to stow gear.

Some wooden 2x4 bridges allow for easier travel across the lush, boggy areas near the streams. Soon, you encounter a series of streams lined with willows and tall, spring-fed wildflowers, where a small pond sits on a bench about 150 feet above the trail. Away from the lush surroundings, you pass through drier foliage to where the trail divides into upper and lower forks.

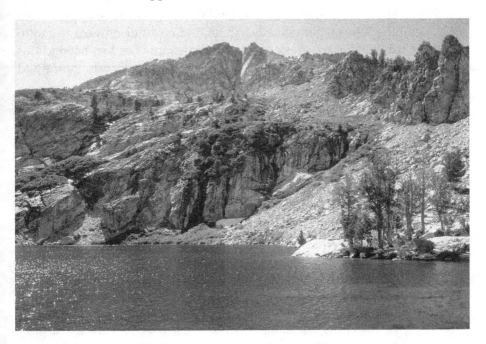

Overland Lake, Ruby Mountains

Tip: *Although the lower route is more direct, the upper route leads over rocky terrain to a beautiful waterfall accented by an impressive display of wildflowers.*

By Yosemite standards, this waterfall won't turn many heads, but here in the Rubies it's a real gem. Thin ribbons of silvery water glide over vertical slabs before merging into a narrow channel, tumbling and frolicking over boulder steps through a garden of deep-green grass, vivid wildflowers, and pockets of willow. Throw in a stone pagoda and a few bonsai plants and you'd have quite the Japanese garden. If you detect the aroma of onion, it's not because you've been away from real food for too long—wild onion flourishes on the stream banks. The majesty of Overland Falls provides a fine place to linger before the journey beckons you onward, as the next decent place to camp with water nearby is still 11 miles ahead.

As the traverse across the canyon continues, the massive hulk of austere King Peak (named for Clarence) dominates the skyline.

Tip: *If you can afford the extra time for an ascent, the summit of King Peak can be reached relatively easily from the trail.*

You cross a branch of Overland Creek, pass above a spring that empties into a willow-lined channel, and continue onward to another tributary of the creek. A beautiful meadow lies just beyond this creek, carpeted with wildflowers, including paintbrush, lupine and daisy.

The long traverse continues, now through drier foliage beneath rock cliffs to a grassy hillside, and then up a steep ascent through tall grass that leads to a small rock knob, where a couple of switchbacks take you up the crest of a minor ridge. From this vantage point, you have an excellent view of the Overland Creek watershed, including the tiny green dot of Overland Lake.

You climb steeply up the next hillside through limber pines until the grade eventually lessens, and you emerge from the pines onto a grass-covered slope sprinkled with wildflowers. For a while, you wind up and down through steep, rocky cliffs, until meadows resume just before the last branch of Overland Creek.

Warning: *Overland Creek is the last place to get water for the nearly 10-mile journey along the Ruby Crest Trail to the springs above North Furlong Creek. Late in the season this final branch may be dry, so at the previous crossing make sure you fill your bottles and fill your stomach.*

Away from the creek, you climb to a sub-ridge, traverse over to another sub-ridge, and ascend through cliffs and meadows to the initial series of switchbacks leading out of Overland Creek canyon. The trail zigzags up a boulder-covered hillside to a notch, which offers a fine view of the canyon. From the notch, the trail follows an ascending traverse before the switchbacks resume. As the grade increases, the vegetation changes to sagebrush and a smattering of stunted pines, before low sagebrush and scattered wildflowers take over near the crest.

The steep climb abates as you approach the summit of peak 10,297, and you gain the crest of the Ruby Mountains. The view of massive, multi-spired King Peak towering above Overland Canyon is quite dramatic. Overland Lake, now 2.5 miles away by air and 5 miles by trail, looks extremely small from this perspective. Ruby Valley, with Franklin Lake below and the Ruby Marshes in the distance, lies to the east. Ahead, the craggy summits of the central Rubies emerge into full view, including Ruby Dome, at 11,387 feet the highest peak in the range. More immediate is the dry ridge that

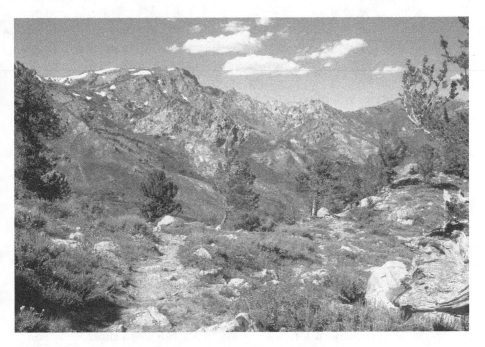

Kings Peak as seen from the Ruby Crest Trail

the trail follows for the next several miles, culminating at Wines Peak, which, despite its romantic appellation is a rather undistinguished hummock.

Now descending, you follow the trail around a hillside and into a saddle. Past the saddle, a gentle ascent heads across the west face of peak 10,394 through sparse, low-growing vegetation, where the tallest thing around is an occasional lupine. Where the grade levels, just below the crest, a sign marked LONG CANYON points downslope to the west.

> **Tip:** Although there is no well-defined path from the Ruby Crest Trail into Long Canyon, by descending the steep hillside you can find water in the creek below. By going all the way to the floor of the canyon, you can intersect the Long Canyon Trail and proceed 6 miles to the Long Canyon trailhead, which is the first exit from the Ruby Crest Trail by maintained trail that does not cross private land.

For the next few miles, the Ruby Crest Trail stays close to the crest of the range, alternately climbing and descending over minor summits and around peaklets from one saddle to the next, occasionally with the aid of switchbacks. The low-growing, sparse vegetation has remained constant since exiting the canyon of Overland Creek. Expansive views to the west and east have been regular features as well. About 10 miles from Overland Lake, from the base of Wines Peak you follow four short switchbacks up the side of the mountain, where views are somewhat occluded by the mass of the peak. A short scramble from the trail up to the summit leads you to a superb view of the central Ruby Mountains.

Descending steeply from Wines Peak, you follow seven switchbacks to a gentler descent on the north side of the mountain toward the upper canyon of North Furlong Creek. Near the bottom, you pass a sign, cross a small seasonal stream, and proceed a short distance to the signed junction with the Furlong Creek Trail, 12.5 miles from Overland Lake. Nearby, you'll find a campsite in a grove of limber pines.

Side Trip to Furlong Lake: Leaving the Ruby Crest Trail, head down the mildly sloping upper canyon across a lush, open basin dotted with wildflowers. The trail may be indistinct in places, but the way is clear and the location of the lake, in a large basin rimmed by steep cliffs, is easy to determine. Occasional cairns may help you to stay on track. The trail draws near to the inviting creek for a while,

Wines Peak

The peak, named for early rancher Ira D. Wines, is visually a rather unimpressive mountain, but it does derive a certain stature from being the highest point along the Ruby Crest Trail, as well as the southern guardian of the Ruby Lakes.

meandering through green meadows before veering away to avoid a willow thicket. Eventually, you follow the trail to a crossing of the creek and head across a good-sized flat above the north shore of the lake, where the path all but disappears. However, from here you'll find the route is obvious over to North Furlong Lake, 0.9 mile from the junction.

The kidney-shaped lake lies at the base of the steep, gray cliffs of Wines Peak, which is a much more impressive sight from this vantage than from the Ruby Crest Trail. A dense stand of limber pine rises up from the south shore. A large green meadow at the west end adds a pastoral ambience to the views down the canyon, which are especially fine around sunset. The lake lacks a permanent outlet, but a delightful little inlet stream cascades from the upper basin and gurgles down a narrow channel that slices through verdant meadows before emptying into the lake.

Backpackers in search of campsites will find some near the south shore and in the meadows west of the lake. A flat above the lake to the north could accommodate large parties. Firewood is relatively plentiful. The shallow lake (20 feet) offers relatively warm water for swimming, but the muddy bottom may be a deterrent for some. Fishing is even less enticing, as brook trout, present in most of the Ruby Lakes, are absent in North Furlong. Despite these minor drawbacks, the excellent scenery and solitude provide a fine haven for backpackers weary from the long hike from Overland Lake. **End of Side Trip**

From the junction with the North Furlong Creek Trail, the Ruby Crest Trail proceeds 0.5 mile up to a pass on the ridge dividing the North Furlong Creek and Kleckner Creek canyons, where you have a fine view of the next canyon, towered over by peaks of the central Rubies. The Ruby Lakes are hidden from view behind the massive slopes of peak 10,468.

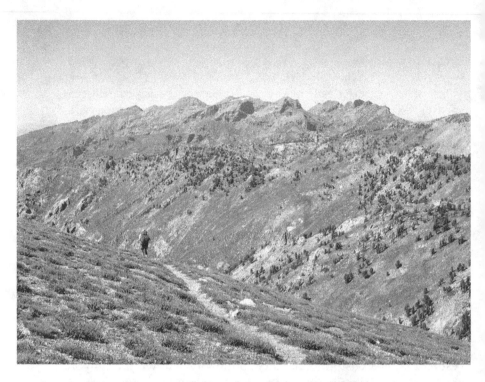

View of the central Ruby Mountains from the Ruby Crest Trail

You follow the trail on a zigzagging descent down the austere, boulder-strewn slopes of the upper canyon, before clumps of limber pine and a sprinkling of wildflowers soften the bleak surroundings. Lower down, the trees grow thicker and taller, wildflowers become more prolific, and pockets of verdant meadow contrast nicely with the large boulders. Paintbrush, asters, bluebells, buttercups, lupine, yarrow, and wild onion are among the species present in the canyon.

After a mile of descent, the grade eases and you round a hillside into a large, open basin and over to a crossing of Kleckner Creek, 2.25 miles from the North Furlong junction. At the crossing, an old use-trail follows the creek upstream a short distance to Favre Lake.

Favre Lake, at 9500 feet, sits in a broad, open bowl at the head of Kleckner Creek canyon, surrounded by green, sloping hillsides that gently dip toward the lake. The rugged, gray cliffs along the north ridge of Lake Peak highlight the limber-pine-carpeted hillside above the southeast shore. Pockets of willow may prevent anglers from capturing the brook trout inhabiting the lake, although access is good on the east side. Despite the fine stand of limber pine shading pleasant campsites along the south shore, firewood is scarce.

Side Trip to Castle Lake: Although a defined trail up to Castle Lake is nonexistent, the route is straightforward and only 0.25-mile long. A usetrail from the south shore of Favre Lake climbs the steep hillside up to the lip of the basin, where the grade mellows considerably. Another 0.1 mile of easy hiking leads to the north shore.

Castle Lake is a delightful place to spend a couple of hours or a couple of days. Carved out of a steep, horseshoe-shaped basin and flanked by the precipitous cliffs of Lake Peak, Castle Lake has much more of an alpine flavor than pastoral Favre Lake. Patches of snow cling to crevices in the gray rock walls of Lake Peak well into summer, adding to the alpine atmosphere. The shoreline is embraced by meadows dotted with willows, with occasional stands of limber pine inching their way up the lower slopes of the basin. Backpackers will find campsites at the north end near the outlet. Unlike at Favre, firewood should be in good supply. Don't unpack your fishing pole, as according to the Forest Service, there are no fish in this lake. However, the little bit of effort involved in reaching Castle Lake should reap extra dividends in solitude. **End of Side Trip**

From Kleckner Creek, you begin the moderate climb toward Liberty Lake, reaching a lateral to Favre Lake after 0.2 mile. From the junction, you angle up the hillside to a switchback and continue the steady ascent to the junction with the short path to Liberty Lake, 1.25 miles from Kleckner Creek.

Liberty is the quintessential mountain lake, with splendid scenery and excellent views. Cradled in a steep-walled basin of rock, perched high above the surrounding canyon, you can appreciate the relative popularity of this lake. Ironically, travelers along Interstate 80, a mere 30 air miles away, race past the range completely unaware of its tremendous beauty, assuming Nevada is nothing more than endless sagebrush and brown-tinged mountains. Campsites are plentiful but firewood is not—be sure to bring a stove if you want hot food or drink. Fishing is good for brook trout.

Warning: The fragile ecosystem around the lake requires that you observe minimum-impact techniques while camping.

From the junction with the path to Liberty Lake, you climb above the steep cliffs to the west of the lake to a viewpoint, where a profusion of wildflowers fills the nooks and crannies amid large boulders. A short, gently ascending traverse leads above the north side of the lake, before the stiff climb toward the pass resumes. A series of switchbacks take you to Liberty Pass (10,400'±), at the signed wilderness boundary. The pass is a cold, windswept, austere, rocky notch, where a few stunted limber pines, some grasses, and a smattering of wildflowers struggle to eke out an existence. None of the lakes behind or ahead of you are visible from the pass, and to the south a string of mountains spreads out along the crest, including Lake and Wines peaks; to the north you gaze down into Lamoille Canyon to Roads End trailhead at the end of Lamoille Canyon Road, where tiny figures scurry around like ants. Three miles of trail is all that separates you from those tiny figures.

The trail winds down from the pass through barren terrain of rock, boulders and slabs, where only a few tiny plants seem capable of surviving the harsh conditions.

Warning: Patches of snow will most likely be on parts of the trail below the pass in early season, and may even cover the path entirely after a particularly heavy winter. Before your trip, check with the Forest Service for current conditions.

Switchbacking steeply down the desolate terrain, you reach an overlook, where Lamoille Lake springs into view, still quite a distance below. After nearly another mile of stiff descent, the grade eases just before a junction with the short lateral to the lake.

Lamoille Lake is cradled in a deep gouge near the west edge of the upper canyon. The steep walls at the head of the canyon rising up towards Liberty Pass make the lake seem rugged and forbidding. The treeless shore appears almost lifeless, but willow brush and grasses thrive in the alpine-like environment. A few campsites are scattered around the north shore, but most visitors coming from Roads End seem content with just a brief visit—hikers enjoy a picnic lunch, and anglers ply the waters in search of brook trout.

Resuming the descent, you head gently downhill past Dollar Lakes, where clumps of willow and green meadows soften the shorelines, and are backdropped nicely by rugged cliffs. You cross the outlet from Dollar Lakes on a crude wooden bridge, gain a hill, and then follow a stiff descent through lush slopes covered with willows and wildflowers to a thick stand of limber pines. You make

several stream crossings before you leave the trees for good, following the verdant slopes down to the parking lot.

POSSIBLE ITINERARY

	Camp	Miles	Elevation Gain
Day 1	South Fork Smith Creek	8.0	1750
Day 2	Overland Lake	6.0	2575
Day 3	Castle Lake	14.0	4375
Day 4	Out	5.5	1000

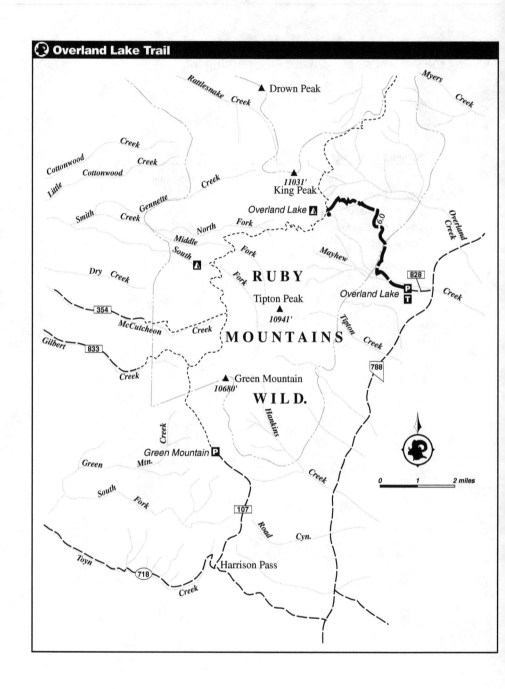

Drown Peak

Myers Creek

Rattlesnake Creek

Cottonwood Creek

Little Cottonwood

Creek

Creek

Creek

Smith Creek

Gennette Creek

11031'
King Peak

Overland Lake 🏕

6.0

Overland Creek

North Fork

Middle

South

Fork

Mayhew

Dry Creek

Fork

RUBY

Tipton Peak
▲
10941'

Overland Lake 🅿🚻

828

Creek

354

McCutcheon Creek

Tipton Creek

Gilbert

833

MOUNTAINS

Creek

788

▲ Green Mountain
10680'

WILD.

Hankins

Creek

Green Creek

Green Mtn.

Green Mountain 🅿

Creek

South Fork

107

Cyn.

Road

0 1 2 miles

Toyn

718

Harrison Pass

Creek

Overland Lake Trail

RATINGS (1–10)			MILES	ELEVATION GAIN	DAYS	SHUTTLE MILEAGE
Scenery	Solitude	Difficulty				
9	10	9	12	3300	2–3	N/A

AREA Ruby Mountains

MAPS USGS-*Franklin Lake NW*; USFS-*Ruby Mountains and East Humboldt Wildernesses*

USUALLY OPEN Late-June to mid-October

BEST July to August

PERMITS None

CONTACT Humboldt National Forest (775) 738-5171

SPECIAL ATTRACTIONS Lake, wildflowers, scenery, views

PROBLEMS Hot and shadeless climb

HOW TO GET THERE The trailhead is off State Route 767, on the east side of the Ruby Mountains. Follow State Route 229, either 36 miles southeast from Interstate 80 exit No. 321, signed HALLECK, RUBY VALLEY, or 14 miles west from U.S. 93, to the junction of 229 and 767.

On 767 follow asphalt highway for 2 miles until the surface changes to gravel. Drive on the gravel road, crossing over Overland Creek at 14.5 miles, until you reach a junction with a dirt road, 1.4 miles farther. A sign at the junction reads simply HUMBOLDT NATIONAL FOREST ACCESS. As you head west toward the mountains another sign on a barbed-wire fence reads OVERLAND LAKE TRAIL. If you miss the turnoff and reach Rock House, you've gone 0.8 mile too far.

If you're concerned about the ability of your vehicle to negotiate the road, park in the grassy area to the left and hike up the road to the trailhead. With a high-clearance vehicle, you can proceed 0.5

mile to the Forest Service gate and park nearby. Off-road 4WD vehicles can continue even farther, to a small knoll where the earth has been bermed to prevent further vehicular progress.

INTRODUCTION The Overland Lake Trail is the only practical route for reaching the heart of the Ruby Mountains from the east side. However, an unrelenting 6-mile climb, beginning near the floor of Ruby Valley, is the price to be paid for that access. Gaining over 3000 feet in the process, backpackers must endure the stiff, shadeless climb across open high desert terrain almost all the way to the lake.

Overland Lake, with a spectacularly beautiful setting perched just below the crest of the range near the head of Overland Creek canyon, is worth the effort. The picturesque lakeshore offers some of the best camping and fishing in the Ruby Mountains Wilderness. For those who don't have the time to complete the Ruby Crest Trail (see Trip 12, p. 137), a weekend excursion to Overland Lake is a fine alternative.

DESCRIPTION From the Forest Service gate, begin hiking up the dirt road over dry, grassy hillsides to the knoll where an earth berm blocks further vehicle progress. Soon the road dwindles to a single-track trail, quickly crossing the wilderness boundary. You continue the steady ascent, winding through sagebrush and grasslands, where views toward the mountains reveal verdant slopes of green foliage and rugged peaks with snow clinging to the cracks and crevices, a definite counterpoint to the typically hot and dry conditions of the foothills.

Eventually, you wind up to a small saddle and pass some interesting rock formations. Above these outcrops, the vegetation transitions to sagebrush and shrubs, interspersed with wildflowers and scattered groves of aspen. A series of switchbacks, followed by a long traverse, leads you to the edge of the canyon, where you have a grand view of the crest across the deep chasm of the Overland Creek drainage. This splendid scene is closer to the type of terrain one associates with mountains, steep canyons, rushing streams, lush vegetation, and jagged peaks.

The trail continues at an unrelenting grade over open slopes, broken only occasionally by groves of aspen. Beyond a seasonal swale, you begin another series of switchbacks, starting a long, zigzagging ascent that ultimately brings you to a junction with the

Ruby Crest Trail, 5.75 miles from the trailhead.

From the junction, turn left and head up a series of eight short switchbacks across a boulder-strewn slope dotted with scattered limber pines. As you reach the lip of the lake basin, the grade eases and you stroll over to the lakeshore near an old cabin, 0.4 mile from the junction.

Overland Lake is an oval body of clear, green-tinged water occupying a

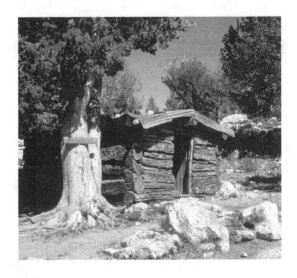

Old cabin near Overland Lake

rugged bowl just below the crest of the range, where talus slopes and rock slabs rise up to steep gray and tan peaks rimming the basin on three sides. Limber pines gracefully add a dose of character to the shoreline. Swimming in the chilly waters will be refreshing on a hot summer day, and fishing for brook trout should be good. Although lightly used, Overland Lake is a common stop for parties hiking the Ruby Crest Trail (see Trip 12, p. 137).

A few campsites are available near the cabin, but the best site is west of the outlet beneath some tall pines. Most equestrians tether their horses on the east side of the creek and set up camp a good distance downstream—hopefully this practice will continue. Firewood is extremely scarce.

Unlike many other geographical features in the Rubies, this lake wasn't named for a settler, but for the Overland Farm, which supplied feed to the horses of the Overland Mail Company 1860s. The old cabin at the north end of the lake looks old enough to have some history as well, but it is of fairly recent origin, used by modern-day horse packers to stow gear.

POSSIBLE ITINERARY

	Camp	Miles	Elevation Gain
Day 1	Overland Lake	6.0	3200
Day 2	Out	6.0	100

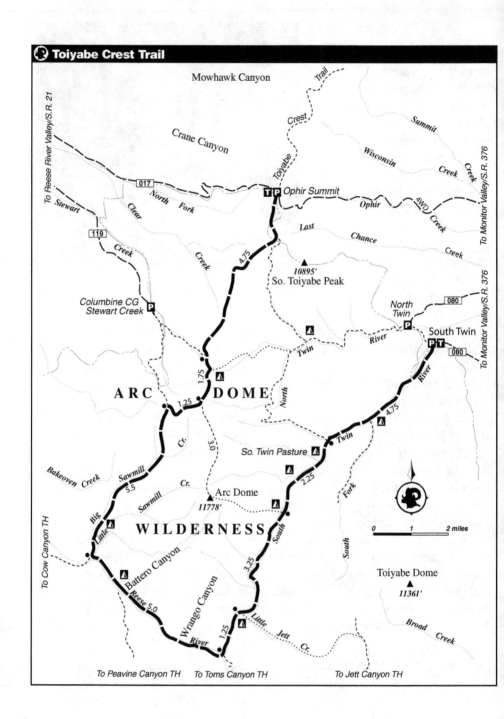

Mowhawk Canyon

Crane Canyon

Trail

Crest

Toiyabe

017

North Fork

Clear

Stewart

119

Creek

Creek

4.75

To Reese River Valley/S.R. 21

TP Ophir Summit

Summit

Wisconsin

Creek

Creek

Ophir

AWD Creek

To Monitor Valley/S.R. 376

Last

Chance

Creek

▲
10895'
So. Toiyabe Peak

Columbine CG
Stewart Creek P

North
Twin

080

P

To Monitor Valley/S.R. 376

1.75

▲

South Twin

PT

080

ARC

1.25

DOME

North

Twin

River

River

4.75

▲

Cr.

3.0

So. Twin Pasture ▲

Twin

▲

2.25

Bakeoven Creek

Sawmill
5.5

Cr.

Sawmill

Cr.

Arc Dome
▲
11778'

▲

Big

Little

▲

WILDERNESS

South

Fork

South

0   1   2 miles

Battero Canyon

Reese 5.0

Wrango Canyon

3.25

Toiyabe Dome
▲
11361'

River

1.25

Little

▲

Jett

Cr.

Broad   Creek

To Cow Canyon TH

To Peavine Canyon TH   To Toms Canyon TH   To Jett Canyon TH

15 Toiyabe Crest Trail

RATINGS (1–10)			MILES	ELEVATION GAIN	DAYS	SHUTTLE MILEAGE
Scenery	Solitude	Difficulty				
8	10	7	30 (+6)	8325 (+1925)	3–5	100

AREA Toiyabe Mountains

MAPS USGS-*Carvers NW, South Toiyabe Peak, Arc Dome, Bakeoven Creek*

USUALLY OPEN Mid-June to mid-October

BEST July

PERMITS None

CONTACT Austin Ranger District (775) 964-2671

SPECIAL ATTRACTIONS Scenery, views, solitude

PROBLEMS Long car shuttle, cattle, lack of campsites, indistinct sections of trail

HOW TO GET THERE *START:* The turnoff from State Route 376, signed SOUTH TWIN RIVER TRAILHEAD, is approximately 40 miles south of U.S. 50 and 61 miles north of U.S. 6. From the junction of S.R. 376 and FS 080, travel northwest on single-lane gravel road (FS 080), passable to sedans, 3 miles to the trailhead. Parking is available in a wide turnout on the south side of the road.

END: The Ophir Creek Road traverses the Toiyabe Range near the north end of the Arc Dome Wilderness, but is impassable to most vehicles from the east, requiring a long drive around the range to complete the car shuttle from the west. A high-clearance vehicle is necessary to reach the Ophir Summit trailhead.

On the Reese River Valley Road, which parallels the Toiyabe Range on the west, drive as far as the Reese River Guard Station, approximately 25 miles south of Highway 50. Just south of the guard station, near the school, turn east onto Forest Service Road 017, signed STEWART CREEK 10, CLEAR CREEK 1, OPHIR WASH 7, CRANE CREEK 5, MOHAWK CANYON 6. Follow gravel road across the Reese River to a Y-junction, 0.4 mile from the Reese River Valley Road, and remain on FS 017, following a sign for OPHIR WASH, MOHAWK CANYON, CRANE CANYON. Remain on the main road (FS 017) at 0.7 mile, where FS 118 branches left.

Ignoring lesser roads at 3.2 and 5.1 miles, you continue on FS 017 past a pair of signs warning NARROW STEEP ROAD and TRAVEL NOT ADVISED FOR LESS THAN ALL WHEEL DRIVE VEHICLES. The road does indeed narrow and the track gets rougher as the grade becomes steeper. At 10.25 miles you pass an old mine, and 0.5 mile farther gain the crest at Ophir Summit. Trail signs may be missing, but the Toiyabe Crest Trail heads south along the twin tracks of an old road. Parking at Ophir Summit is limited to a couple of vehicles, but that seems more than adequate for the amount of use this trailhead receives.

INTRODUCTION The Toiyabe Crest Trail is the highlight of any venture into the Toiyabe Mountains. Although the entire trail is 66 miles in length, only the first 30 are within the Arc Dome Wilderness, and the description that follows covers only that initial segment. Outside the wilderness, the path is truly a "crest" trail, traveling along the spine of the Toiyabes from the edge of the wilderness to Kingston Canyon. Within the Arc Dome Wilderness, the trail initially avoids the top of the range, following the South Twin and Reese rivers on a horseshoe bend before adopting a northbound course that climbs along the crest for the last 7 miles to Ophir Summit.

Passing through terrain between roughly 6000 and 11,000 feet in elevation, the Toiyabe Crest Trail exposes backpackers to a wide range of environments. Sampling lush riparian foliage along three major drainages, travelers will experience a diverse mixture of trees, shrubs, and wildflowers. Along these streams, a relatively small amount of water transforms the high desert into a luxuriant display of foliage. Significant stands of aspen fill some of the higher canyons, putting on a dramatic display of color during autumn. Above the streams, pinyon-pine-juniper woodland adorns the lower slopes, intermixed with the characteristic sagebrush. Higher up, limber pines grace the hillsides along the upper canyons and

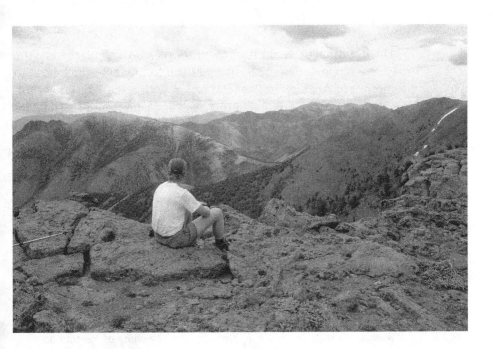

View from the Toiyabe Crest

ridgecrests. On the 11,000-foot plateau near Arc Dome, you'll see that low sagebrush and alpine-like flora soften the otherwise austere surroundings.

The Toiyabe Crest Trail was a Civilian Conservation Corps work project during the 1930s. Unfortunately, due to its obscurity and a lack of proper funding, the trail has not received the care and attention that the original builders probably would have liked. Although rarely maintained, the path remains in fair condition and is relatively easy to follow for most of the way through the Arc Dome Wilderness, except at a couple of obscure junctions. However, these junctions along with some other sections of faint trail shouldn't present any insurmountable route finding problems for anyone able to understand a topographic map.

While the first few miles of trail are moderately steep, somewhat brushy, and require numerous fords of the South Twin River, the middle section is through the wide-open, rolling terrain of the Reese River country. Anyone vaguely familiar with old western movies can easily imagine a posse of white hats pursuing a band of cattle rustlers through the open terrain. Anglers will appreciate some of the best fishing in the state.

The trail then turns up Big Sawmill Creek on a climb toward the top of the range, where peak baggers can follow a 3-mile lateral to the summit of Arc Dome. The last section within the Wilderness follows the crest of the range to a dirt road at Ophir Summit. The one-way trip will require a lengthy car shuttle between the South Twin River and Ophir Summit trailheads.

If you plan on completing the entire 66-mile length of the Toiyabe Crest Trail, be aware that the section outside the Arc Dome Wilderness is dry, requiring that backpackers descend into side canyons to find water from springs and streams. Early in the season, lingering snow banks may provide an easier way to get water. Although this trail corridor is technically outside the Arc Dome Wilderness, the Forest Service manages it as de facto wilderness, closed to motorized travel.

DESCRIPTION

Warning: Despite the initial impression, the beginning of the trail does not follow the continuation of the mining road up the canyon alongside the river, but instead follows a single-track trail that cuts diagonally across the hillside in the opposite direction. The road, built in 1980 to provide access to a mining claim up the river, fords the stream numerous times in the first 0.75 mile, and is almost impossible to follow on foot without getting your feet soaked.

From the trailhead, follow the trail across the hillside to a switchback, and continue to climb steeply through pinyon pine, sagebrush, and ephedra toward a cluster of sharp cliffs. After cresting the first rise, follow gently-descending trail to rejoin the mining road coming up from below, and then climb up to the top of another knoll, 0.9 mile from the trailhead. A remarkable vista unfolds down into the deep cleft of the canyon, which is enclosed by steep walls and dramatic cliffs. While taking in this remarkable scene, you can't help but wonder how the South Twin River ever managed to carve its way through the maze of cliffs at the entrance to the canyon.

Following the road, you descend through pinyon-pine-juniper woodland to the floor of the canyon. The grade eases as the path comes alongside the river, and you stroll through willows, alders, and cottonwoods. As the rocky road continues upstream, wild rose, currant, chokecherry, and desert peach join the riparian vegetation alongside the river, along with a variety of wildflowers, including columbine, paintbrush, lupine, bluebell, and penstemon.

Having avoided the lower fords along the mining road, you now must ford the river several times before arriving at the site of a relic, an old mill wheel that utilized water power to process ore from a nearby mine. Past the mill, the old road crosses the river, passes a campsite, quickly fords the river again and reaches a junction with a trail heading up the South Fork, 3.5 miles from the trailhead.

Tip: For parties getting a late start, a passable campsite is just 50 feet up the South Fork trail

From the junction, a single-track trail now follows the course of the South Twin River through lush riparian foliage, including cottonwoods, wild roses, and grasses. More fords await, as you climb alongside the river to a signed junction with the North Twin River Trail, 4.75 miles from the trailhead, where a primitive campsite is nearby.

Just below the junction, the canyon widens and the steep rock walls give way to sloping, sagebrush-covered hillsides. Gently graded trail leads away from the junction 0.75 mile to South Twin Pasture, a broad, moist meadow. Pleasant campsites will tempt you to overnight here, as long as you don't have to share your spot with the cattle that occasionally graze in this part of the canyon.

Beyond the half-mile-long meadow, the grade increases as you climb up the east bank of the diminishing river, reaching a side canyon on the opposite side, 0.25 mile past South Twin Pasture, where you'll find a delightful campsite near a seasonal creek. A faint use-trail follows the course of this canyon up toward the summit of Arc Dome.

You continue along the narrow river up the canyon, where sagebrush covers the hillsides and aspen lines the streambed. Where the trail crosses the river, the fords become easier thanks to the lessening flow. Above the sea of sagebrush, scattered limber pines start to show themselves in the upper canyon. The summit of Arc Dome makes a brief appearance through the broad gash of a canyon to the west as you reach a crudely signed junction with an unmaintained trail to the summit, 7 miles from the trailhead. The old sign indicates a distance of 2.5 miles to the top.

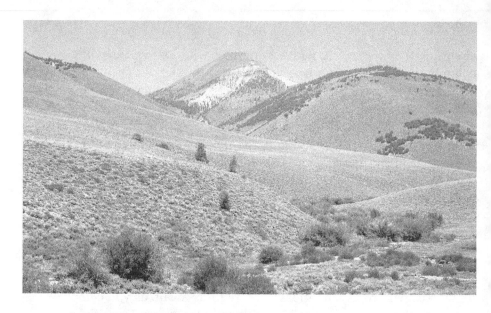

Arc Dome from Toiyabe Crest Trail

Proceed from the junction on soft dirt tread, through grasses and sagebrush. Limber pines and aspens cover the hillsides in the upper canyon, where a sprinkling of lupine adds a delightful touch of blue in early summer. The grade increases as you ascend toward the divide that separates the South Twin River and Reese River watersheds. At 7.75 miles, you arrive at the grassy pass in a grove of mountain mahogany accented by widely scattered limber pines. The broad basin of the upper Reese River spreads out before you. The rolling hills carpeted with silvery-green sagebrush and the endless sky bring to mind a cowboy country image—the only missing piece is John Wayne astride his stallion.

From the pass, the Toiyabe Crest Trail follows a gradual, continuous 9-mile descent to the confluence with Big Sawmill Creek. Through dwarf limber pine, you descend to the floor of the wide-open canyon to the crossing of the trickling headwaters of the Reese River. The lightly used path is lost for a time in the grass of the upper canyon, but the way down the gorge is clear and there is more distinct tread farther downstream.

You cross a side stream, where Arc Dome briefly returns to view, and then ascend a low hill before the path comes alongside the river again. Proceed downstream, crossing the river a few times before your arrival at Little Jett Canyon, 10.25 miles from the trailhead. Just below some beaver ponds, you can ford the river to campsites in a grove of tall aspens alongside Little Jett Creek. Even if you don't plan on spending the night, this relaxing spot is well suited for a rest stop. Nearby, a fairly well-defined trail, marked by a sign reading JETT CANYON, runs along the creek and heads up the canyon toward the ridge dividing Little Jett and Jett canyons.

For the next 1.25 miles, the path wanders between grassy meadows and fields of sagebrush, crossing the river once before reaching the signed junction with the Toms Canyon Trail, 11.5 miles from the trailhead. By midsummer, Trail Creek is usually bone dry.

Cross the swale of Trail Creek into thick brush, as the trail bends west to follow the course of the Reese River. Asters and daisies have joined the retinue of wildflowers growing amid the streamside vegetation. Soon the trail crosses over to the north bank and veers away from the river through sagebrush and rabbitbrush. Beavers have lived up to their reputation of being busy by building a number of dams and ponds along this stretch of the river. You follow the trail across a gravel bar, ford the river, and then head over more gravel to a meadow.

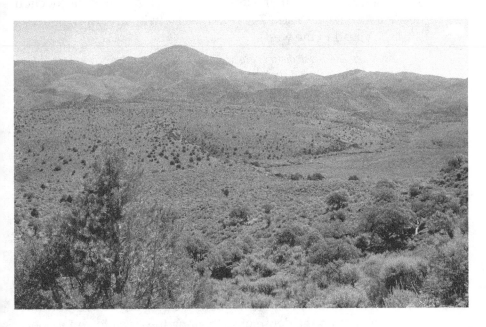

Arc Dome and the Reese River country, Toiyabe Range

Continuing the mild descent, you make several river crossings over the next few miles, most of which present little problem to negotiate. However, the fifth crossing after the meadow occurs in the backwater of a beaver dam, requiring you to wade through a relatively deep pool of water, even in late summer.

You follow the trail on a brief climb above the steep declivity of Wrango Canyon before descending back alongside the river. Eventually, the path follows a fenceline leading to a large camp area on the north side of the river, where widely spaced aspens provide filtered shade for campsites in a patch of grass, complete with fire pits and sitting logs. A private corral used by horse packers is across the river, as well as a connection with the Peavine Canyon Trail.

From the camp, you quickly pass a smaller campsite, this one complete with outhouse. Two more fords of the river and a steep climb bring you to the mouth of Battero Canyon, where for the first time in a long while you have a view of Arc Dome. Another 1.25 miles brings you to an easy crossing of Little Sawmill Creek. A short distance beyond the crossing, 5 miles past the Toms Canyon junction and just before Big Sawmill Creek, you come to a somewhat confusing junction with the Reese River Trail. A sign at the junction reads BIG SAWMILL CREEK, 7 STEWART CREEK (with an arrow pointing straight ahead to the west).

Warning: *The most distinct tread does indeed continue straight ahead across the creek, but that path is the Reese River Trail.*

To continue on the Toiyabe Crest Trail, turn 90 degrees north, pass through an opening in a barbed-wire fence, and head up the east side of Big Sawmill Creek. The faint path eventually becomes more distinct as you continue upstream.

The lush vegetation of the slender canyon immediately strikes you, where sagebrush, rabbitbrush, and wild rose cover the ground below quaking aspen. A profusion of wildflowers, including columbine, primrose, and lupine, adds splashes of color. Soon, the trail leads you across Big Sawmill Creek to ascend the west bank between low cliffs and through thick riparian foliage to a small grassy clearing. At this point, rocky cliffs force the trail back to the east side, as willows and alders choke the stream banks. Now the trail returns to the west side, where the canyon widens and then veers away from the dense growth along the creek to a more open hillside. Arc Dome, hidden for some time, now becomes an intermittently seen companion, looming high above the surrounding terrain.

As you approach a pyramidal rock, the trail bends down to the creek again to avoid steep cliffs on the west side of the canyon. Under the shade of mature aspens, a wide flat offers a nice campsite near the stream. A short distance up the trail, 1.6 miles past the junction, a glade of aspen holds an even better campsite, with fire pits, sitting logs, and a gated livestock corral.

Once again the trail veers away from the creek,

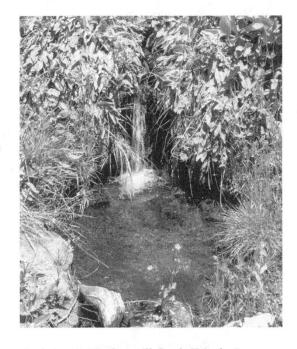

Spring near Big Sawmill Creek, Toiyabe Range

passing through typical sagebrush-covered slopes. As you enter the upper part of the canyon, the gorge narrows and the walls get steeper, and the trail alternates between the lush riparian foliage along the creek and the drier vegetation of the hillsides. As you proceed upstream, mountain mahogany and limber pine become more prolific. At 3.5 miles from the Reese River Trail junction, you cross the main branch of Big Sawmill Creek.

After the crossing, you climb well above the level of the tributary stream, across a sagebrush-covered hillside. A moderately steep ascent leads to a small gorge, where an aspen-lined rivulet provides a brief respite from the laborious climb. Follow the trail back into the main canyon and travel high above the stream, until the trail and the creek nearly converge for a brief stint higher up the canyon. Now you climb above a grassy, spring-fed meadow to the top of a rise, where the trail disappears in the open grassland. Cairns should guide you across this clearing to the resumption of defined tread. Impressive views to the west include the Shoshone Mountains and distant ranges beyond. After crossing a dry swale, you make a gentle climb to an unmarked junction with the

Columbine Jeep Trail (see Trip 16, p. 171), 5.5 miles from the Reese River Trail junction.

Continue on the Toiyabe Crest Trail, which angles back sharply from the junction to climb steeply southeast up the track of the old jeep road, with the aid of some switchbacks. You pass through low-growing sagebrush and grasses to easier hiking on the plateau at the crest of the range, where sections of faint tread are aided by the placement of occasional ducks and cairns. After hiking 1.25 miles along the old jeep road, you reach the junction with the trail to Arc Dome.

> **Tip:** *The trail to Arc Dome heads south for 3 miles to the 11,773-foot summit, gaining 1350 feet and losing 625 feet along the way. Views from the top are quite rewarding; the whole of Arc Dome Wilderness with its peaks and canyons lies at your feet, while the mountains of the Toquima, Monitor, and Shoshone ranges are in the near distance. On clear days, the outline of the Sierra Nevada is visible to the west, over 100 miles away.*

From the Arc Dome junction, the trail bends northeast, and after 0.25 mile leaves the crest to drop into the upper canyon of a tributary of the North Twin River. A 0.75-mile descent brings you to a junction with a path that heads down the tributary. For those in search of water or a passable campsite, a brief climb, incorporating three short switchbacks, takes you to a high, windswept saddle along the crest, followed by a half-mile descent through limber pines and shrubs to the unsigned junction with the Stewart Creek Trail, 1.75 miles from the Arc Dome junction (see Trip 17, p. 177).

As you head away from the junction on a moderate climb back to the crest, the lush foliage thriving in the Stewart Creek canyon stands in vivid contrast to the struggling vegetation along the exposed ridge. From the top of a minor peak, you have an excellent view of the northern section of Arc Dome Wilderness. A more gradual climb along the crest takes you over the shoulder of the next peak. Large cairns appear periodically, despite the good condition of the trail (they would have been much more valuable in the trail-less sections of the previous canyons). A high traverse around the shoulder of a ridge leads to a gradual descent to a notch in the crest, where you are afforded excellent views of the surrounding topography, including the impressive cliffs of the North Twin River canyon.

From the notch, a descent wraps around the shoulder of the mountain and back to the crest again, where low-growing sagebrush, scattered wildflowers, and an occasional limber pine cling to the slopes below volcanic outcroppings. You traverse northwest around the backside of a ridge until a moderately steep climb takes you up to a minor crest. A mild descent then leads to a descending traverse of another hillside through mature limber pines over to another saddle.

You ascend mildly until the grade increases near a grove of mountain mahogany on a winding ascent to the top of a sub-ridge, followed by a brief descent to a long traverse around the west side of the crest, proceeding through low sagebrush and sporadic limber pines. At the end of the traverse, a short but exceedingly steep climb leads across the ridge and to a saddle and a junction with an obscure trail, 5 miles from the trail to Arc Dome.

From the saddle, you make an ascending traverse above the canyon of Last Chance Creek and then climb steeply to another saddle along the crest. Another traverse along the west side of a minor peak provides unobstructed views across Reese River Valley to the Shoshone Mountains and distant ranges. After ascending a short rise, the Ophir Creek Road springs into view, and you follow a twin-tracked jeep road to the trailhead, 6.5 miles from the Arc Dome junction.

Warning: *The Toiyabe Crest National Scenic Trail continues another 35 miles to Kingston Canyon, remaining near the crest for most of that distance. Unfortunately, the trail lies wholly outside of Arc Dome Wilderness, and water is hard to come by, particularly after snowmelt.*

POSSIBLE ITINERARY

	Camp	Miles	Elevation Gain
Day 1	Little Jett Creek	10.25	3250
Day 2	Big Sawmill Creek	8.0	500
Day 3	Out	10.25	4575

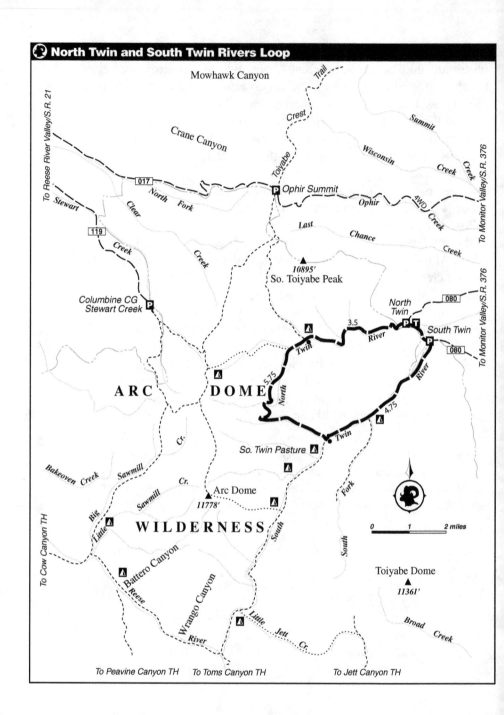

Mowhawk Canyon

Crane Canyon

To Reese River Valley/S.R. 21

Crest

Trail

Summit

Toiyabe

Wisconsin

Creek

Creek

To Monitor Valley/S.R. 376

017

North Fork

Ophir Summit

Ophir

Last Chance

4WD Creek

Creek

Clear

Stewart

119

Creek

Creek

10895'
So. Toiyabe Peak

Columbine CG
Stewart Creek

North Twin

080

3.5
River

South Twin

080

To Monitor Valley/S.R. 376

ARC

DOME

5.75

North Twin

River

4.75

So. Twin Pasture

Twin

Cr.

Bakeoven Creek

Sawmill

Cr.

Sawmill

Big

Arc Dome
11778'

Fork

South

0   1   2 miles

Little

WILDERNESS

South

Battero Canyon

Toiyabe Dome
11361'

Reese

Wrango Canyon

Little

Jett

Cr.

Broad Creek

River

To Cow Canyon TH

To Peavine Canyon TH   To Toms Canyon TH   To Jett Canyon TH

16

North Twin and South Twin Rivers Loop

RATINGS (1–10)			MILES	ELEVATION GAIN	DAYS	SHUTTLE MILEAGE
Scenery	Solitude	Difficulty				
7	9	6	14	3475	2	1

AREA Toiyabe Mountains

MAPS USGS-*Arc Dome, Carvers NW, South Toiyabe Peak*

USUALLY OPEN Mid-June to mid-October

BEST July

PERMITS None

CONTACT Austin Ranger District (775) 964-2671

SPECIAL ATTRACTIONS Canyon scenery, solitude

PROBLEMS Frequent river crossings

HOW TO GET THERE *START:* Following a sign marked NORTH TWIN RIVER, turn west from State Route 376 in Smoky Valley onto Forest Service Road 080, approximately 37.5 miles south of U.S. 50 and 63 miles north of U.S. 6. Drive on single-track gravel road, passing into Toiyabe National Forest at 2.3 miles, to an intersection with the road to the South Twin trailhead at 3.5 miles from the junction. Continue straight ahead another 0.3 mile to the trailhead, where you'll find parking for only a few cars. If space is not available, park in a large area near a pile of boulders about 50 yards back down the road.

END: The North Twin and South Twin trailheads are just 1 mile apart, accessible on foot via an old dirt road that requires a ford of the South Twin River, which normally just gets your feet wet, but in early season may present a formidable challenge.

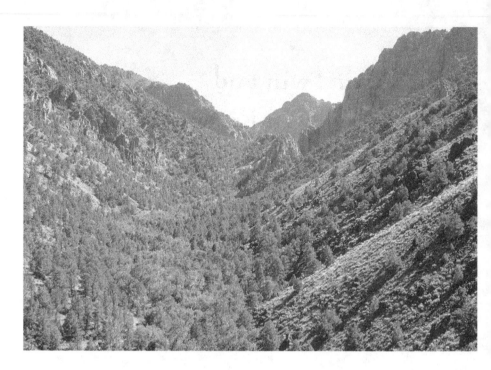

South Twin River canyon, Toiyabe Range

To reach the South Twin trailhead with a vehicle, the turnoff, signed SOUTH TWIN RIVER, is 2.6 miles south of the turnoff for the North Twin trailhead. Follow the single-lane gravel road 3 miles to the wide turnout on the south side of the road.

INTRODUCTION Only by Nevada standards can these two streams be referred to as rivers, but what the North Twin and South Twin rivers lack in volume, they certainly make up for in vibrancy, drama, and wonder. These twins share a family resemblance, both winding down narrow gorges, overshadowed by towering cliffs rising abruptly from the valley floor and piercing the deep blue sky with jagged pinnacles and serrated ridges. Also, both streams roar down their respective canyons in resounding cacophony, through numerous cascades, swirling pools, and churning cataracts.

Subtle differences between the two canyons do reveal themselves during the course of the loop. North Twin flows down a narrower canyon, while taller and more interesting cliffs appear in the canyon of South Twin. While both rivers support healthy riparian vegetation along their banks, particularly in the lower reaches of the canyons, North Twin holds the lusher environment. With their similarities and differences, the North and South Twin rivers are two precious siblings, highlights of the Arc Dome Wilderness.

Early in the season, especially following winters of heavy snowfall, the route is potentially dangerous, as hikers are forced to make numerous crossings of both streams. Contact the Forest Service for current conditions. Even in low-water conditions, packing along a pair of tennis shoes or sandals for the various fords is a wise idea. With so many opportunities to slip off a wet rock into the roaring stream, even the most adroit hiker can't expect to beat the law of averages.

After the first couple of miles beyond the mouths of the canyons, the problem resolves, as the ravines tend to widen enough to allow the trail to stay on one side of the river for extended periods, and the lower volume of water allows easier fords.

Although more or less limited to the sites mentioned in the description, campsites occur at strategic locations and are generally quite pleasant. Opportunities for further exploration abound, including off-trail routes to the summit of Arc Dome.

DESCRIPTION Starting at the wilderness boundary, the North Twin River Trail follows the river as it winds upstream through cottonwoods, junipers, and pinyon pines. As forewarned, the trail quickly comes to a ford of the river, a process repeated around 15 times within the first 2 miles. The path weaves back and forth through the narrow, twisting canyon, as the river tumbles and churns on a precipitous course toward a more placid course on the floor of Big Smoky Valley.

Beyond the first couple of miles, the canyon widens and the grade eases as the river glides alongside banks lined with pinyon pine, willow, and wild rose. The canyon narrows again for a short time around a stand of aspen, but you quickly break out into the open surroundings of a meadow. Beyond the meadow, the lush riparian foliage becomes quite dense. After another river crossing, you emerge into an extensive, aspen-filled meadow. Nearby is the signed trail junction with the Ophir Creek Trail, 3.5 miles from the trailhead, where a faint track ascends a side canyon to the northwest past Werdenhoff Pasture. Campsites near the junction under the shade of mature aspens provide a fine place to lay your head for the night, providing cattle haven't arrived here before you.

For the next 0.6 mile, you wander through dense aspen and thick underbrush, crossing the river several more times, to an unsigned junction with a path ascending the next side canyon.

After the unmarked junction, you cross the river, hop across a side stream, and enter open slopes above the river filled with sagebrush and other shrubs. Indian paintbrush and lupine add a splash of color in early summer. Eventually, the trail returns to the riparian vegetation near a flat along the river, where you'll find a pair of small campsites alongside a seasonal side stream, 4.5 miles from the trailhead.

Now the trail forsakes the river as you climb away in earnest, initially through aspens and then across exposed, sagebrush-covered hillsides. An array of wildflowers complement the gray-green hue of the sagebrush, including lupine, paintbrush, and bluebells. Farther up the slopes, scattered groves of mountain mahogany offer pitiful amounts of shade as you climb steadily toward the top of the ridge. In the midst of your climb, a very brief descent leads to a small stream, which turns out to be the thin ribbon of upper North Twin River, coursing through a gully. Away from the nascent stream, the ascent continues and you pass through a significant stand of aspen and limber pine before reaching the top of the grassy divide, 6 miles from the trailhead. A grove of mountain mahogany provides just enough shade for a relaxing break, as you enjoy the fine view of the surrounding canyons and peaks.

Away from the pass, you descend fairly steeply through thick mahogany sprinkled with a smattering of limber pine into a canyon, through which flows a tributary of the South Twin River. You follow the creek downstream across sagebrush-covered slopes to where the drier vegetation alternates with lush foliage near the stream. After traversing a long talus slope, the path follows tradition by crossing the creek several times. Toward the bottom of the canyon, cottonwoods, willows, and wild roses begin to reappear along the banks of the stream, while the slopes above continue to be covered with sagebrush and mountain mahogany. Just before the confluence of the South Twin River, you follow the trail through a grassy meadow, cross the stream one last time, and come to a signed junction with the South Twin River Trail, 8.25 miles from the trailhead. Campsites can be found 0.4 mile upstream at South Twin Pasture.

As you head downstream, you may notice that the vegetation in the South Twin River canyon is drier than its counterpart, as pinyon pine covers the slopes, along with some juniper and even sparser limber pine. Heading northeast, you follow the course of the river, making numerous crossings as the canyon deepens and dramatic cliffs tower over the agitated water. At 1.4 miles from the junction, you encounter another junction, this one with the trail up the South Fork. A fairly decent campsite is a short distance from the junction up the South Fork.

Now you follow an old mining road, which is extremely rocky in places, and wander across the river, above the river, and along the banks in a seemingly arbitrary fashion. Where impressive rock cliffs seem to bar the river's escape from this canyon, you begin a steep climb heading for the top of an outcrop. At the top of the climb, a dramatic view of the canyon awaits.

From the outcrop, the old road makes a curving descent toward the bottom of the canyon and the river, but you should avoid going that way, as the road makes numerous crossings of the river that would thwart the nimblest of hikers. Instead, head along the hillside on single-track trail to the next rise of cliffs. You climb up through pinyon pine, sagebrush, and ephedra, over the cliffs, and then make a half-mile descent to the trailhead.

If you don't have a vehicle at the South Twin River trailhead, you'll have to ford the South Twin River and follow the old road back to the North Twin trailhead.

POSSIBLE ITINERARY

	Camp	Miles	Elevation Gain
Day 1	North Fork Twin River	4.5	2175
Day 2	Out	9.5	1300

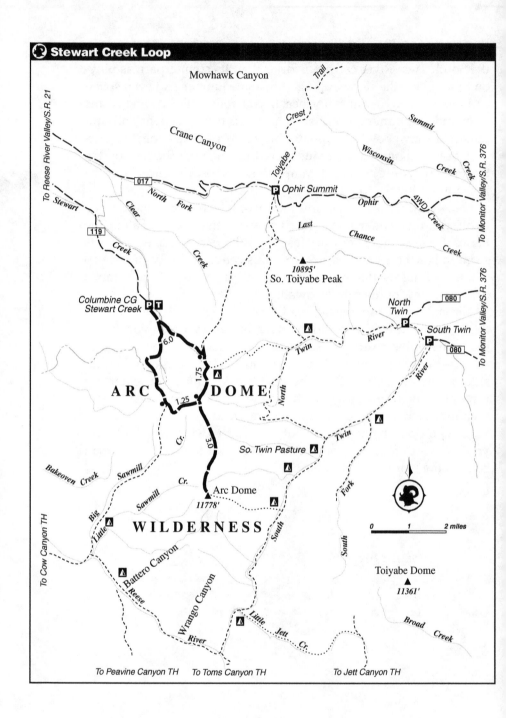

Mowhawk Canyon

Trail

Crest

Summit

Crane Canyon

Toiyabe

Wisconsin

Creek

Creek

To Reese River Valley/S.R. 21

017

North   Fork

Ophir Summit

Ophir

4WD Creek

To Monitor Valley/S.R. 376

119

Clear

Stewart

Creek

Creek

Last   Chance   Creek

10895'
So. Toiyabe Peak

Columbine CG
Stewart Creek

North
Twin

080

South Twin

To Monitor Valley/S.R. 376

6.0

1.75

River

Twin   River

080

ARC   DOME

North

1.25

Twin

3.0

Cr.

So. Twin Pasture

Bakeoven Creek

Sawmill

Fork

Cr.

Sawmill

Arc Dome
11778'

Big

WILDERNESS

South

South

To Cow Canyon TH

Little

0   1   2 miles

Battero Canyon

Toiyabe Dome

11361'

Reese

Wrango Canyon

River

Little   Jett   Cr.

Broad   Creek

17 Stewart Creek Loop

RATINGS (1–10)			MILES	ELEVATION GAIN	DAYS	SHUTTLE MILEAGE
Scenery	Solitude	Difficulty				
8	9	8	9 (+6)	2675 (+1925)	2–3	N/A

AREA Toiyabe Mountains

MAPS USGS-*Arc Dome, Bakeoven Creek, Corral Wash, South Toiyabe Peak*

USUALLY OPEN Mid-June to mid-October

BEST July

PERMITS None

CONTACT Austin Ranger District (775) 964-2671

SPECIAL ATTRACTIONS Canyon scenery, solitude, views, wildflowers

PROBLEMS Indistinct sections of trail, poor campsites

HOW TO GET THERE Drive the Reese River Valley Road to the junction with FS Road 017, just south of the Reese River Guard Station and the school. For the duration of your drive to the trailhead, follow all signs labeled STEWART CREEK. Head east on 017, crossing over the Reese River at 0.1 mile, and proceed to a Y-junction with FS Road 119 at 0.4 mile. Turn right onto 119 and continue to a Y-junction at 1.0 mile from Reese River Road, where you bear right, cross Clear Creek, and quickly come to another Y-junction. Bear left at this junction and proceed to yet one more Y-junction at 1.6 miles from the Reese River Road, where you turn to the right.

Near a fenceline, 2.7 miles from the Reese River Road, bear to the right at a junction. Farther on, near a sign marked TOIYABE NATIONAL FOREST, follow the main road to the right, crossing Stewart Creek at 5.7 miles, and then continue on FS Road 119 east for 3 more miles into the narrowing, aspen-lined canyon of Stewart Creek. At 8.7 miles, you drive past a horse-loading area and a lateral trail used by horse packers marked TOIYABE CREST TRAIL. Continue on the main road over a cattle guard and into Columbine Campground, 9 miles from the Reese River Road.

A sign for CREST TRAIL on the right-hand side of the road near a pole gate designates the hikers' trailhead. Parking is available around the campground loop road for about half a dozen vehicles.

INTRODUCTION Columbine is one of the nicest Forest Service campgrounds in the Nevada system, a wonderful setting for a night's rest after the long drive. Two different routes branch off from a junction just 0.25 mile from the campground, providing an opportunity for an excellent loop that passes through a diverse set of environments. Add in a climb to the summit of Arc Dome, the highest peak in the Toiyabe Range at 11,773 feet, and you have the makings of a fine adventure.

The first part of the loop climbs steeply through one of the most luxuriant stream settings in central Nevada; thick stands of aspen fill the Stewart Creek canyon from one side to the other, offering a swath of green in summer and a blaze of gold in autumn. Along with the aspens, an abundance of wildflowers graces the hillsides and a profusion of riparian foliage lines the banks. At the head of the canyon near the Toiyabe Crest, majestic limber pines cover the slopes.

Two miles above the campground, the Stewart Creek Trail meets the Toiyabe Crest Trail, where the loop heads south toward an 11,000-foot-high plateau, providing spectacular vistas in every direction. On the plateau, a 3-mile trail branches away from the Crest Trail toward the summit of Arc Dome, where even more dramatic views await.

Dropping off the crest, the loop takes you across sagebrush-covered slopes, with more fine views back into the Stewart Creek drainage, and past an expansive meadow before returning to the lush vegetation of the lower canyon.

Developed campsites are few and hard to come by away from the lower sections of Stewart Creek, but the scenery won't disappoint you.

DESCRIPTION Follow the track of the old jeep road from the campground, through aspens, shrubs, and wildflowers, soon breaking out into the open to views of the upper canyon. After 150 yards, you reenter aspen cover and quickly arrive at a junction, 0.25 mile from the campground. The jeep road, the return route of the loop, continues to the right, heading south toward a connection with the Toiyabe Crest Trail near the headwaters of Sawmill Creek. Veer left onto single-track trail following a sign for STEWART CREEK TRAIL, TOIYABE CREST TRAIL ½ (the .5 mile is wildly inaccurate—2 miles is closer to the actual distance).

You head through thick brush and aspen to a crossing of Stewart Creek, and then wind uphill amid lush plants and shrubs, wildflowers, and more aspens to a minor ridge, where you momentarily break out into the open. Climb along the crest of this ridge, which separates two forks of the creek, and quickly come back under the filtered shade of light aspen cover. Briefly back out in the open again, dramatic views of the Reese River Valley and the Shoshone Mountains stretch out behind you to the west.

After cresting a small knoll in a sea of sagebrush dotted with wildflowers the grade eases, but only for a short time. Across a small, grassy meadow carpeted with flowers and ringed by aspens, a bewildering sign, marked TOIYABE CREST TRAIL (with an arrow to the left) and N. TWIN RIVER 5, BIG SAWMILL CREEK 4 (with an arrow to the right), seems to indicate a trail to the south, but thick foliage has obscured any trace of a trail, offering no clues to the mysterious junction, which is also absent from the USGS map.

As you continue east up the drainage through dense vegetation, a more defined track reappears beyond the meadow. Where the canyon starts to narrow and limber pine and mountain mahogany make an appearance, you cross the creek to the north bank and begin a steeper climb with the aid of some switchbacks. After passing some weather instruments, you climb steeply to the unsigned junction with the Toiyabe Crest Trail, approximately 300 feet below the crest of the range, 2.25 miles from the campground.

From the junction, you turn south and climb 0.4 mile through low-growing shrubs and scattered limber pine to a saddle along the crest. From there, three short switchbacks lead to a signed junction with a trail descending east down a tributary of the North Twin River to water and campsites.

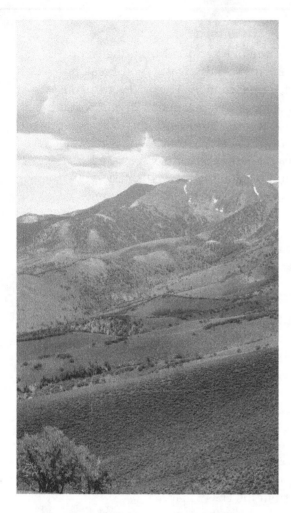

A short traverse leads into the swale of a seasonal drainage, which the trail follows steeply to a low gap at the edge of a broad plateau near 11,000 feet, where Arc Dome dominates the skyline immediately to the south. You reach a junction with the trail to the summit of Arc Dome, 1.75 miles from the junction between the Stewart Creek and Toiyabe Crest trails.

Tip: The trail to Arc Dome heads south for 3 miles to the 11,773-foot summit, gaining 1350 feet and losing 625 feet along the way. Views from the top are quite rewarding; the whole of Arc Dome Wilderness with its peaks and canyons lies at your feet, while the mountains of the Toquima, Monitor, and Shoshone Ranges are in the near distance. On clear days, the outline of the Sierra Nevada is visible to the west, over 100 miles away.

A thunderstorm brews over Arc Dome

You descend west across the mildly sloping plateau before a steeper descent along an old jeep road leads you across a sagebrush-covered hillside to an unmarked junction between the Toiyabe Crest and the Columbine Jeep trails, about 1.25 miles from the Arc Dome junction.

The Crest Trail bends sharply south toward the canyon of Big Sawmill Creek, but you continue straight ahead on the jeep road, winding down the hillside with Reese River Valley and the Shoshone Mountains in full view to the west. As the path slices across the hillside, a large green meadow springs into view below. After circling around some cliffs, the trail leads down to a crossing of Stewart Creek, where the luxuriant foliage lining the banks is almost overwhelming after the drier vegetation along the crest.

Follow the east bank of the creek to the expansive meadow. If it weren't for the fence around the perimeter and the usual herd of grazing cattle, this meadowland would be a stunning wilderness scene. On gently graded trail, pass just above the east edge of the clearing to a gate at the far end of the meadowland, before a stiff descent resumes through sagebrush, grasses, and wildflowers. Soon, dense stands of aspen fill the lower part of Stewart Creek Canyon, and you pass the signed junction with the obscure lateral to the Stewart Creek Trail. Descend to a crossing of the west branch of the creek and across a sloping meadow above the far bank, which holds a couple of little-used campsites. Through dense foliage, you reach the junction with the Stewart Creek Trail, 2.6 miles from the junction with the Toiyabe Crest Trail. Continue the final 0.25 mile back down to Columbine Campground.

POSSIBLE ITINERARY

	Camp	Miles	Elevation Gain
Day 1	North Twin Tributary	3.25	1975
Day 2	Out	5.75	700
+	Side trip to Arc Dome	6.0	1925

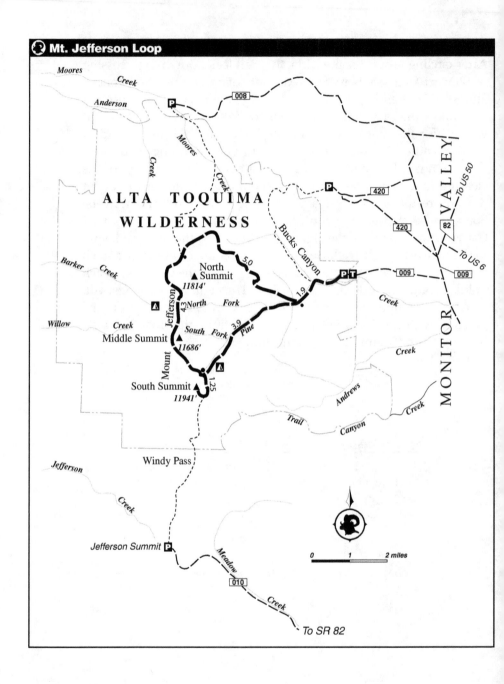

18   Mt. Jefferson Loop

RATINGS (1–10)			MILES	ELEVATION GAIN	DAYS	SHUTTLE MILEAGE
Scenery	Solitude	Difficulty				
8	10	7	17 (+2.5)	5475 (+1075)	2–3	N/A

AREA Toquima Range

MAPS USGS-*Pine Creek Ranch, Mt. Jefferson*

USUALLY OPEN Mid-June to mid-October

BEST Late June to July

PERMITS None

CONTACT Austin Ranger District (775) 964-2671

SPECIAL ATTRACTIONS Scenery, views, solitude, alpine flora

PROBLEMS Indistinct sections of trail, lack of campsites, rattlesnakes in lower canyon

HOW TO GET THERE Drive on the Monitor Valley Road (Secondary Road 82) to the junction with Pine Creek Road (FS 009), approximately 57 miles south of U.S. 50 and 47 miles north of S.R. 376. Head south on 009 for almost a mile to a junction, where you bear right. Near the 3-mile mark, you cross into Forest Service land and continue to the Pine Creek Campground, 3.5 miles from the Monitor Valley Road. Campsites are straight ahead, while the trailhead is just up a short road to the right, in a wide clearing immediately north of the campground.

INTRODUCTION The seldom-seen topography in the Alta Toquima Wilderness has much to offer both the casual recreationist and the serious nature lover. Beginning in juniper-pinyon pine woodland, hikers quickly encounter lush riparian foliage along the lower

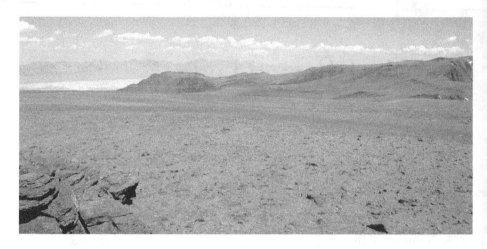

The plateau on top of Mt. Jefferson

reaches of tumbling Pine Creek. Aspens and limber pines are dominant on the upper slopes of the canyon, until desert-alpine vegetation takes over at the summit of Mt. Jefferson.

Nearing the crest, the Pine Creek Trail intersects the Mt. Jefferson Trail, which runs north-south along the crest of the triple-summited massif. South Summit, highest of the three and Nevada's sixth highest summit at 11,941 feet, has a short, technically easy route from the trail to the top, where a supreme vista awaits. North of South Summit, the trail climbs onto the Mt. Jefferson plateau, a long, narrow tableland looming over glaciated side canyons, passing directly below Middle Summit before skirting well to the west of North Summit. The gentle topography along the plateau allows for easy hiking, and the low-growing, alpine vegetation permits excellent vistas from one horizon to the other.

The route eventually leaves the crest to descend into remote Bucks Canyon before cresting over a saddle and returning to Pine Creek. Although discernible trail is lacking over parts of the route, the cross-country hiking is not particularly difficult.

DESCRIPTION Away from the trailhead, the Pine Creek Trail follows the continuation of the old road for a short distance until bending uphill, where a single-track trail veers away to the left. Quickly, you pass a use-trail coming in from the campground, then step over a seasonal stream and immediately reach the wilderness boundary. Over the next half-mile, you cross the densely-foliated creek three times before encountering a junction with the Pasco Canyon Trail, 1.2 miles from the trailhead.

Continue up the Pine Creek Trail through lush riparian foliage, crossing the creek several more times, before arriving at an obscure junction with the trail heading northwest up Bucks Canyon, 1.9 miles from the trailhead. This faint path will ultimately provide your return to the trailhead.

The trail up the canyon continues to wander back and forth over the creek. Near one of these crossings, approximately 3.75 miles into the journey, you pass an acceptable campsite. Under the shade of aspens, you wind upstream amid grasses and wildflowers for a considerable distance until an open area of sagebrush allows sweeping views of the upper canyon. Near the 4-mile mark, you follow the trail across the narrowing creek to a spring-fed meadow, where the trail temporarily disappears in the tall grass.

Beyond the meadow you pick up the discernible tread of a rocky path and start to climb more steeply in and out of the filtered shade of aspens and limber pines.

Tip: By midsummer, parts of the creek in the upper canyon may be dry, but a spring 4.5 miles from the trailhead will provide ample water. This may be your last water source until Bucks Canyon, so be sure to fill all your containers.

You leave the limber pines behind just beyond the spring and steeply ascend grassy slopes to the last crossing of the streambed, just below where a couple of small springs send a trickle of water into the swale. Now you ascend the wide-open upper canyon, where grassy meadows meld into the austere terrain of the rock-covered slopes. The trail, which has been in remarkably good condition up to this point, disappears in the meadow grass; look for ducks to guide you to a distinct junction with the Mt. Jefferson Trail, 5.8 miles from the trailhead. A large cairn marks the junction along with a sign supported by a weathered tree limb that reads S. SUMMIT, (left) NORTH SUMMIT (right).

Side Trip to South Summit: Turn left (southeast) from the junction and climb across a talus slope to the top of a ridge, where you encounter the faint trace of a path heading down Andrews Creek and over to Windy Pass. Bear west from the ridge and make a steep ascent across the east face of South Summit to the crest of the southeast ridge. Leave the trail and head up easy slopes to the top, 1.25 miles from the Pine Creek Trail junction. The 360-degree view from South Summit is quite a reward for the short climb. **End of Side Trip**

From the Pine Creek Trail junction, turn left (northwest) and continue up the final slope of the canyon to the low point on the crest above. As you ascend out of the Pine Creek basin, the trail fades away, but ducks will guide you past cliffs to where the path becomes distinct again. Following a switchback, the trail curves around to gain the crest and then disappears once more.

Now the long plateau atop Mt. Jefferson stretches out before you, where desert-alpine vegetation struggles to attain heights of even 3 to 4 inches, and wildflower blooms are short-lived. Awe-inspiring, 360-degree views are commonplace, with mountains from California to Utah visible on clear days. Across Big Smoky Valley to the west, Arc Dome presides over the Toiyabe Range, and across Monitor Valley to the east sits the vast, mesa of aptly-named Table Mountain.

> *Warning:* *Although maps indicate a defined trail across the length of Mt. Jefferson's plateau, only short sections of the path are the least bit discernible. However, only rudimentary route finding skills are necessary to negotiate the open topography across the gently sloping tableland.*

Once on the crest, the route proceeds for a mile over rising terrain to the rocks just below Middle Summit, by far the easiest of the three peaks to scale. From Middle Summit, the pseudo-trail heads along the crest for another 1.25 miles before a mild descent brings you to a large meadow, where the USGS map indicates the presence of a perennial stream, the beginning of Barker Creek. Unfortunately, the stream on the map is more like a wet bog on the ground; don't plan on acquiring water here, especially if cattle are present.

Beyond the meadow, you make a short ascent to a saddle directly east of point 11215, from where distinct tread descends into the Barker Creek drainage—a good option if you're in search of a campsite or water. The main trail veers to the right and climbs steeply up a rocky hillside to milder slopes above. Having regained the top of the plateau, the path heads north to what at one time may have been an actual junction with the trail descending east toward Bucks Canyon.

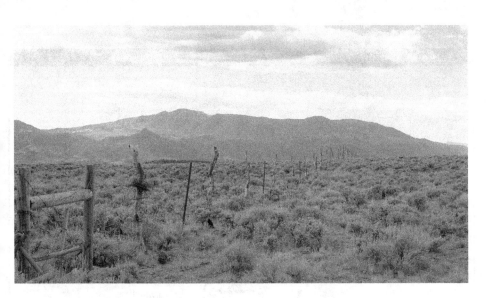

Toquima Range from Monitor Valley

At the old junction, 4.25 miles from the junction with the Pine Creek Trail, you leave the Mt. Jefferson Trail, head east to Peak 11691, and continue along the rocky ridge, keeping a watchful eye out for the most promising way down the precipitous slope into Bucks Canyon. Once the difficult part of the descent from the ridge into Bucks Canyon is over, you should be able to find the faint trace of a path that leads to a crossing of the stream, and then, after a brief climb out of the canyon, follows a mildly descending traverse across the slopes below North Summit to a saddle. From the saddle, you drop into the canyon of a tributary of Pine Creek and descend along the stream to the main channel and a reunion with the distinct Pine Creek Trail. From there, retrace your steps 1.9 miles to the trailhead.

POSSIBLE ITINERARY

	Camp	Miles	Elevation Gain
Day 1	Upper Barker Creek	9.5	4325
+	Side trip to South Summit	2.5	1075
Day 2	Out	7.5	1150

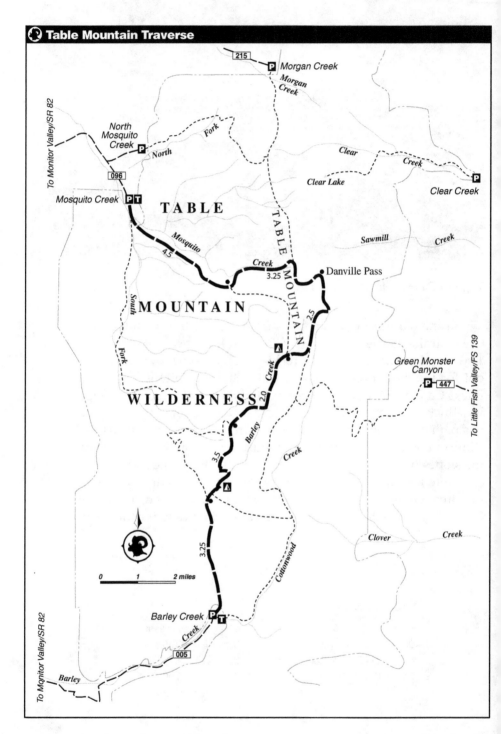

215

P Morgan Creek

Morgan Creek

North Mosquito Creek P

North

Fork

Clear

Creek

To Monitor Valley/SR 82

096

Mosquito Creek P T

TABLE

Mosquito
4.5

Clear Lake

P

Clear Creek

Sawmill

Creek

Creek
3.25

Danville Pass

MOUNTAIN

South

Fork

2.5

WILDERNESS

Creek

2.0

Green Monster Canyon

P 447

To Little Fish Valley/FS 139

Barley

3.5

Creek

Clover

Creek

0 1 2 miles

3.25

Cottonwood

To Monitor Valley/SR 82

Barley Creek P T

Creek

005

Barley

19 Table Mountain Traverse

RATINGS (1–10)			MILES	ELEVATION GAIN	DAYS	SHUTTLE MILEAGE
Scenery	Solitude	Difficulty				
8	10	7	19	2975	2–3	32

AREA Monitor Range

MAPS USGS-*Mosquito Creek, Danville, Green Monster Canyon, Barley Creek*

USUALLY OPEN Mid-June to mid-October

BEST Late June through July

PERMITS None

CONTACT Austin Ranger District (775) 964-2671

SPECIAL ATTRACTIONS Scenery, views, solitude, fauna and flora

PROBLEMS Indistinct and missing sections of trail

HOW TO GET THERE *START:* Drive on the Monitor Valley Road (Secondary Road 82) to the junction with the Barley Creek Road (FS 005), about 70 miles south of U.S. 50 and 34 miles north of State Route 376. Head east across Monitor Valley on well-graded road to a major intersection. Following signed directions for S FORK BARLEY CREEK 1, BARLEY CREEK 2, COTTONWOOD CREEK 4, you turn right onto narrower and rougher road and travel 1.5 miles to a T-junction. Turn left at the junction and proceed 0.4 mile to another T-junction, marked BARLEY CREEK RANCH ½ (left) COTTONWOOD CREEK 4 (right). Basically, the route has made a detour around the private property of the Barley Creek Ranch.

Turn right at the junction and proceed northeast on FS 005 up the canyon of Barley Creek, crossing the stream four times before reaching a broad turnaround at the trailhead, almost 4 miles from the junction with the road to Barley Creek Ranch. On the way up the canyon, you pass numerous primitive campsites, one with a pit toilet nearby. Amenities at the trailhead include a stock-loading area, pit toilet, picnic tables, campsites, and small corral.

END: Drive on the Monitor Valley Road to the intersection with the Morgan Creek-Mosquito Road and travel northeast for 5.75 miles to the junction with FS 096. Turn east onto FS 096, following a sign for MOSQUITO CREEK, and continue 2 miles to the trailhead next to Mosquito Creek. Two fine campsites are near the trailhead underneath some cottonwoods and pinyon pines. The trailhead has a stock-loading area as well.

INTRODUCTION The Table Mountain Wilderness is named for the sloping, roughly rectangular, 12-square-mile plateau along the northern crest of the Monitor Range, home to some of Nevada's largest stands of aspen and to some of the state's most expansive vistas. A thriving population of wildlife and a fine assortment of wildflowers add to the beauty this area has to offer backpackers and other recreationists. Mid-June to mid-July is an excellent time to visit, just when the flowers are at their peak and plenty of water is running in the streams; late September to early October is a grand time to see the aspens at the height of their glory, audibly complemented by the bugling of male elk.

The Barley Creek Trail starts off as a mellow 3.5-mile stroll up the canyon of Barley Creek before steeper terrain must be negotiated on the way up to Table Mountain. Most of the initial terrain is composed primarily of sagebrush-covered hillsides, but after the first 7 miles the prolific stands of aspen come into view. Atop Table Mountain, impressive views open up to the west and east.

Horse packers and equestrians find the mild grade of the Barley Creek Trail especially appealing, and constitute the majority of the limited traffic this trail receives. Like many of the trails within the Wilderness, Barley Creek offers connections to a network of trails that cross Table Mountain, providing opportunities for extended visits into the backcountry. Unfortunately, many sections of trail are hard to follow or gone altogether, and few funds are available to the Humboldt-Toiyabe National Forests for trail maintenance. Anyone planning a visit to the heart of Table Mountain Wilderness should be proficient at navigation and off-trail hiking.

After experiencing the parkland of Table Mountain, your hike proceeds along the Mosquito Creek Trail, following the aspen-lined creek for the first couple of miles before veering away and descending through dry slopes, filled with sagebrush and dotted with pinyon pine, mountain mahogany and juniper.

DESCRIPTION From the well-signed trailhead, follow a new section of single-track trail on a climb across the hillside to a gate and then back to the course of the old road. You proceed up the gently rising roadbed, winding up the canyon below steep, rocky cliffs, crossing the small, willow-lined stream several times along the way. Away from the lush riparian foliage lining the creek, you pass through tall sagebrush and scattered pinyon pines and junipers. You cross the seasonal stream near a small grove of mountain mahogany, where a crude wooden sign reads TABLE MTN 9. Beyond the stream crossing, continue up the canyon on gently graded trail.

Near the 3.25-mile mark is an unsigned, indistinct junction, where the left-hand trail branches away from Barley Creek and heads toward Big Meadow, Dry Lake, and Serpentine Wall. Veering to the right, proceed upstream along the east bank of Barley Creek on a trail that that isn't shown on the USGS map. Just 0.25 mile past the obscure junction, 3.5 miles from the trailhead, you reach a second junction, with a trail heading east that later connects to the Cottonwood Creek Trail. Although the junction is indistinct as well, this path at least has a sign 25 feet from the junction that reads COT-TONWOOD CR. 3.

You start to climb more steeply, passing first a tiny spring and then a grove of quaking aspens, where you see some campsites that seem quite capable of handling several tents. Beyond the camp, the steep climb leads to an area of extensive beaver activity, where numerous dams and ponds have radically altered the terrain in the narrow gorge, with many aspens toppled in the process.

Past the beaver activity, you cross Barley Creek and begin a steep climb up the far hillside toward a gap in the ridge above. Outside the canyon, the lush foliage along the creek is replaced by sagebrush-covered hillsides dotted with widely scattered mahogany, juniper, and pinyon pine. After cresting a rise, you'll see views open up to the west of Mt. Jefferson and the rest of the Toquima Range.

Follow the trail in and out of a couple of minor drainages and continue toward Table Mountain, ascending open slopes carpeted with sagebrush. After passing through an opening in a barbed-wire fence, you reach an unmarked junction with the trail to Dry Lake, 6.75 miles from the trailhead.

Continue straight ahead from the junction, remaining on Barley Creek Trail 038, which follows the course of an old jeep road on a gentle climb toward the top of a rise and then back alongside the upper portion of Barley Creek. You walk along a fenceline to an open gate and continue another 100 yards to a grassy meadow and the crossing of the creek at 8.5 miles. Just beyond the crossing, a path continues upstream to some excellent campsites near a grove of aspen.

The main trail turns away from Barley Creek to follow the course of an old jeep road on a moderately steep ascent up the east wall of the canyon, toward the crest of the Monitor Range. After 0.5 mile, the grade eases and you turn north to make a mild climb near the spine of Table Mountain. A mile farther you reach a junction, where there is a choice of two different routes to Mosquito Creek. The jeep road on your left follows a straightforward, moderate descent toward the stream canyon, while the path straight ahead continues toward Danville Pass before connecting to a trail that descends more steeply into the Mosquito Creek drainage.

From the jeep road, a gently graded, 0.75-mile ascent takes you to the high point of your journey, at 10,640'±, before a steep descent drops to Danville Pass. Table Mountain provides one of the finest parkland experiences in Nevada, with acres of aspen groves and open meadows with incredible vistas.

Tip: Parties with extra time can enjoy much more of Table Mountain by continuing northbound on the Morgan Creek Trail. »

Leave the pass area and head west on a steep descent into the head of the canyon where the southern tributary of Mosquito Creek is born. After about 0.5 mile, the canyon curves to the north and you encounter a junction with the aforementioned jeep road. Beyond the junction, you pass around an aspen grove and follow very indistinct trail down the open hillside to where the two branches of the creek come together and the trail becomes more apparent. At the edge of a meadow, a well-defined trail follows the north tributary 0.75 mile to a connection with the Morgan Creek Trail.

However, you continue downstream through the meadow as the path grows faint again alongside the main channel of Cottonwood Creek. Nailed to one of the first trees at the far edge of the meadow a wooden sign reads MOSQUITO CR TH 7. For the next 1.25 miles, the trail, not shown on the USGS *Mosquito Creek* or *Danville* quad, stays close to the creek, passing through dense aspens, many with some of the largest trunks imaginable. Plenty of inviting campsites are found in the grass beneath the tall trees.

Eventually, you veer away from the creek and head south, following nearly level trail through open slopes of sagebrush, fringed with pockets of aspen running up the hillside. About 2 miles from the previous junction, you reach an unmarked, three-way junction. Turn west and descend past a large stand of aspen back toward the canyon of Mosquito Creek. After a mile you reach the crest of a sub-ridge, from where you have a fine view back up toward Table Mountain, carpeted with expansive stands of aspen. Descend a short vale to the south of the main channel before returning to the canyon of Mosquito Creek, where the trail stays high above the stream, although wandering over to the aspen-lined creek is fairly easy if a refreshing break or a campsite is needed.

The descent continues across a seasonal drainage and across open slopes of sagebrush dotted with an occasional pinyon pine, and you have fine views across Monitor Valley of Mt. Jefferson and the Toquima Range. You continue the moderate descent until steep switchbacks lead down rocky terrain to drier slopes of widely spaced sagebrush, ephedra, juniper, and pinyon pine. After passing the wilderness boundary, you cross Mosquito Creek and reach the trailhead, 4.75 miles from the three-way junction.

POSSIBLE ITINERARY

	Camp	Miles	Elevation Gain
Day 1	Upper Barley Creek	8.5	2275
Day 2	Out	10.5	700

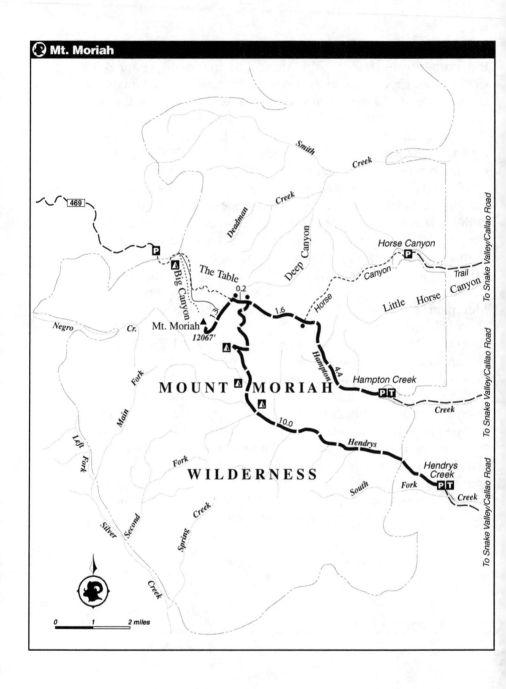

The Table
0.2

Horse Canyon
P

Canyon

Trail

To Snake Valley/Callao Road

Smith

Creek

Creek

Deadman

Deep Canyon

Little Horse Canyon

469
P

Big Canyon

Negro   Cr.   Mt. Moriah
12067'

1.6

Horse

1.3

Hampton

4.4

Hampton Creek
P T

Creek

To Snake Valley/Callao Road

MOUNT   MORIAH

Main

Fork

Left Fork

Fork

WILDERNESS

10.0

Hendrys

Spring Creek

South   Fork

Hendrys
Creek
P T

Creek

To Snake Valley/Callao Road

Silver   Second

Creek

0   1   2 miles

Mt. Moriah

RATINGS (1–10)			MILES	ELEVATION GAIN	DAYS	SHUTTLE MILEAGE
Scenery	Solitude	Difficulty				
9	10	8	16 (+3)	5470 (+1250)	2–3	15

AREA Snake Range

MAPS USGS - *The Cave, Old Mans Canyon, Mt. Moriah*

USUALLY OPEN Mid-June to mid-October

BEST Late June through July

PERMITS None

CONTACT Ely Ranger District (775) 289-3031

SPECIAL ATTRACTIONS Scenery, solitude, views

PROBLEMS Indistinct and missing sections of trail

HOW TO GET THERE *START:* Along U.S. 50, approximately 58 miles east of Ely and 90 miles west of Delta, Utah, is a junction with State Route 487 heading southeast to Baker and to Great Basin National Park. At this junction, turn northeast onto paved Callao Road. After 0.5 mile, a sign reads HENDRYS CREEK 15, HAMPTON CREEK 21, HORSE CREEK 24, SMITH CREEK 28. At 2 miles from U.S. 50, the surface changes to gravel as you pass through the Silver Creek Ranch. You cross the Utah border at 9.3 miles and reach the turnoff for Hendrys Creek 1.4 miles farther, immediately prior to a Y-junction with a prominent gravel road from the south.

Turn northwest onto a narrow dirt road signed HENDRYS CREEK 4, near a concrete headstone and a mailbox reading HATCHROCK, MT. MORIAH STONE INC. Follow the main road, crossing back into Nevada after 1.6 miles, and continuing to a Y-junction at 3.25 miles from the gravel road, where you veer left, following a sign marked TRAILHEAD (the right-hand road heads off into the now-defunct Hatchrock stone quarry).

Proceed through an open gate and cross into National Forest land near the 4-mile mark, quickly reaching the trailhead at a wide, gravel turnaround. A trail sign and register marks the beginning of the trail.

END: From the Hendrys Creek junction, continue northbound on the gravel road another 4.1 miles to the turnoff with the road up Hampton Creek.

Head west toward the mountains on a narrow, rough, dirt road, crossing into National Forest land near the 5.5-mile mark. Follow the road on a stiff climb alongside Hampton Creek, passing several mining operations along the way. At 6.25 miles, you pass a road on the left that heads down toward a small campsite with picnic table and fire ring near the creek, and quickly reach the trailhead, where parking is available for a half dozen vehicles.

INTRODUCTION The highlight of any trip to the Mt. Moriah Wilderness has to be the namesake peak itself. A 10.5-mile hike, followed by a short and easy off-trail scramble, leads to the summit of 12,067-foot Mt. Moriah, Nevada's fifth highest peak, where summiteers are treated to some of the finest views in the region. Adjacent to Mt. Moriah is The Table, a broad, 7000-acre, mildly sloping plateau at 11,000 feet, having a unique environment of alpine plants and wind-battered bristlecone pines. The open topography of The Table affords excellent views of Mt. Moriah and the surrounding terrain. An optional side trip to the Big Canyon cirque on the northeast flank of Mt. Moriah offers additional rugged mountain scenery.

Before the alpine heights in the core of the wilderness can be experienced, backpackers must make the journey up one of the stream canyons that spiral away from Mt. Moriah. This description follows the course of Hendrys Creek to Mt. Moriah, with a return via Hampton Creek, passing through a variety of interesting terrain along the entire length of the trail. Dramatic rust-hued cliffs line the lower canyons, where shrub-covered slopes provide good vistas away from the riparian vegetation along the creek. Farther up the gorges, a healthy mixed forest limits the views, but shades hikers from the intense eastern Nevada sun.

You encounter a wide variety of plant zones along the trail, from pinyon-juniper woodland in the lower canyons to bristlecone pine

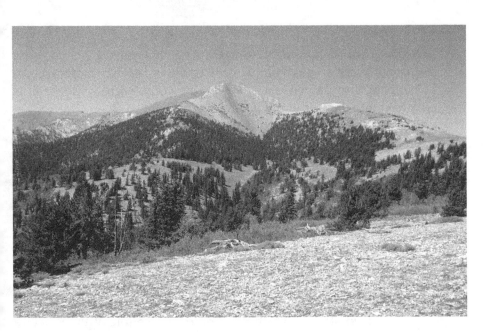

Mt. Moriah from The Table

forest at the highest elevations. In between, ponderosa pines, white firs, Douglas firs, limber pines, and subalpine firs form one of the most diverse coniferous forests in the state. Large stands of quaking aspen along the streams and in the upper canyons provide a sea of light green in summer and a blaze of gold in autumn.

The Snake Range offers some of the most remote backcountry in the West. The vast majority of what little traffic the region does experience is concentrated to the south, in Great Basin National Park. The opportunity for solitude in Mt. Moriah Wilderness is as close to a sure thing as you can get. Anglers should enjoy the opportunity to fish streams that see little pressure. However, this remoteness is not without drawbacks, as trails running through here are infrequently maintained, if at all, and sections of trail that appear on maps may not appear on the ground. Developed campsites are few and far between, but along Hendrys Creek at least, backpackers should fine satisfactory sites.

DESCRIPTION Follow the continuation of the old road alongside the creek. Where the canyon makes a sweeping bend, views reveal steep hillsides rising up to rugged cliffs along the rim of the basin. You drop down to a crossing of the creek, quickly followed by a hop across a spring-fed side stream. On a gently graded path, you pass through scrub oaks complemented by occasional cottonwoods, junipers, and pinyon pines. Where the gorge narrows, the trail is forced into dense cottonwoods along the canyon floor.

Farther upstream, ponderosa pines begin to join the mixed forest, as wild roses and alders mingle with the dominant shrub oaks. You cross over the main creek two more times before reaching the signed wilderness boundary, approximately 1.75 miles into your journey. From the boundary, proceed in and out of light forest beneath dramatic, rust-red cliffs. Quaking aspens, white firs, subalpine firs, and Douglas firs make appearances, ultimately thickening into a fairly dense forest farther up the canyon. Near the site of the old Hendrys sawmill, a stone chimney is all that remains of a former cabin.

Beyond the old mill site, the trail leads you alongside a lovely, flower-lined stream, which you hop over a couple of times before reaching the source at a spring emerging from a low hillside bursting with wildflowers, including columbine, paintbrush, daisy, aster, and shooting star. Where the canyon narrows considerably, you pass through an opening in an old log fence and cross Hendrys Creek amid a mixed forest interspersed with dense groves of aspen. One of those aspen groves harbors a sheltered campsite near an unusual looking piece of iron machinery.

Continue upstream as the V-shaped canyon veers sharply north and the grade of ascent increases. Farther up the slender gorge, three aspen-covered flats, each with a comfortable campsite, interrupt the predominantly coniferous forest, composed mainly of white fir and Douglas fir. You make numerous crossing of the diminishing creek and smaller tributaries on the way to a long, thin, wildflower-carpeted, spring-fed meadow. Across the meadow, you have your first limited views of Mt. Moriah. The fringe of the meadow is a good place to camp, although developed sites are hard to come by.

Beyond the meadow, the trail forsakes the course of the creek, angling back to steeply ascend a hillside covered with limber pine. You gain the crest and follow the ridge, where bristlecone pines become the dominant conifer. The trail veers away from the ridge as you make an ascending traverse across a pair of seasonal drainages and an intervening ridge and then reach a junction with the

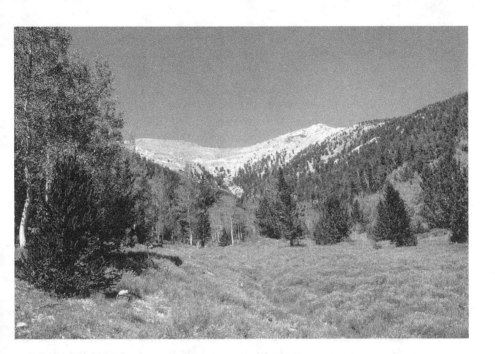

Meadow along Hendrys Creek Trail, northern Snake Range

Hampton Creek Trail on the southeast edge of The Table, 10.0 miles from the trailhead.

Turn west at the junction and follow the faint track of the trail for 0.2 mile to the northeast ridge of Mt. Moriah. Leave the path behind and follow ducks and cairns up a steep slope over the crest of the ridge and along the backside to a saddle, where you should be able to locate a distinct path again. Follow a use-trail on a traverse across the slope below the satellite peak just northeast of the true summit. Continue the general traverse over to a saddle between the two peaks and then across the east face of Mt. Moriah. Inexplicably, the distinct tread falters below the south side of the peak, as if a trail crew had broken for lunch and had never returned, but the remainder of the ascent is easy and uneventful. Views from the summit, in the rarified air of eastern Nevada, are expansive and extraordinary, providing a deep sense of remoteness.

At some point you will have to pull yourself away from the inspiring views and retrace your steps down the northeast ridge back to the trail and over to the junction between the Hampton Creek and Hendrys Creek trails.

Tip: *Parties who won't mind an 1100-foot climb on the return can elect to follow the continuation of the trail eastward down into Big Canyon. The dramatic scenery in the cirque at the head of Big Canyon, below the northeast face of Mt. Moriah, is a near equal to the much more popular cirque below Wheeler Peak in Great Basin National Park. The stream in Big Canyon is intermittent in nature, but if your visit is early enough in the season, a campsite with such scenery combined with available water may be too good to pass up, despite the climb back to The Table.*

Following the Hampton Creek Trail away from the Hendrys Creek Trail junction, you continue across the mildly sloping plateau of The Table, where scattered pockets of contorted bristlecone pine, along with a few Englemann spruce, add character to the wide-ranging views. Short, alpine grasses carpet the floor of the plateau and early-season wildflowers provide a vibrant burst of color. Pieces of trail appear, disappear, and reappear along the route across The Table, but the way is obvious, and periodically placed ducks and cairns will aid your travel. At the far edge of the plateau, you drop through a clearing that provides a farewell glimpse of Mt. Moriah into a light forest of bristlecone pine. Continuing the descent, subalpine firs eventually replace the bristlecones and the trail becomes hard to follow, although more ducks should provide guidance. In a grassy meadow, 1.6 miles from the junction, you encounter the unmarked junction with the primitive Horse Canyon trail.

Beyond the meadow, the trail becomes steeper as the descent along Hampton Creek begins through an extensive grove of aspens, followed by a forest of bristlecone and limber pines. You cross the creek numerous times, shaded by the dense forest that transitions to Douglas firs, white firs, and ponderosa pines, losing more elevation. A series of six switchbacks leads down to a crossing of the creek one more time and out of the mixed forest to drier surroundings, where mountain mahogany becomes the dominant tree.

Quickly back into a mixed forest of aspens, pines and firs, the single-track trail meets an old roadbed, which takes you to an abandoned ditch, used long ago to supply water for a nearby garnet mine. The grade eases beyond the ditch as the road winds around a hillside well above the level of the creek through pinyon-pine-juniper woodland to the wilderness boundary.

Continue down the old roadbed at an increased grade to a section of newer trail that switchbacks down the hillside, rejoining the road a short distance below, where a short, moderate descent leads to the trailhead.

POSSIBLE ITINERARY

	Camp	Miles	Elevation Gain
Day 1	Upper Hendrys Creek	8.5	4220
Day 2	Out	7.5	1250
+	Side trip to Mt. Moriah summit	3.0	1250

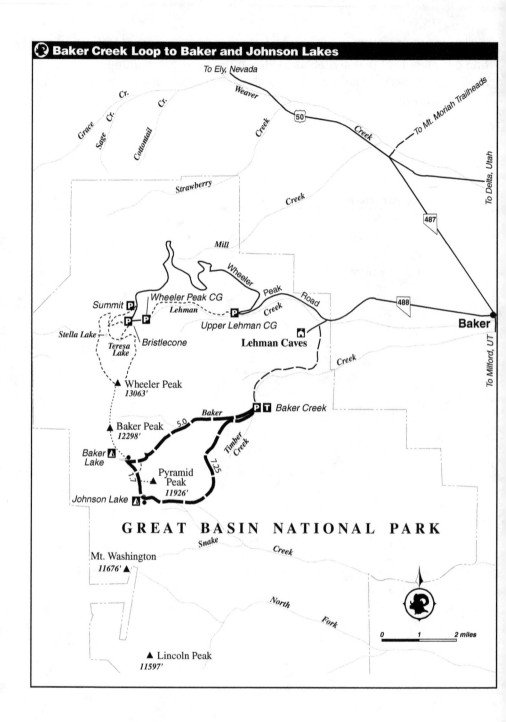

To Ely, Nevada

Weaver

Grace Cr.

Sage Cr.

Cottontail Cr.

Creek

50

Creek

To Mt. Moriah Trailheads

To Delta, Utah

Strawberry

Creek

487

Mill

Wheeler

Peak

Road

488

Baker

Summit P

Wheeler Peak CG

Lehman

P

P

Stella Lake

Teresa
Lake

Bristlecone

P

Upper Lehman CG

Creek

Lehman Caves

Creek

To Milford, UT

Wheeler Peak
13063'

Baker Peak
12298'

Baker
Lake

Baker

5.0

Baker Creek

P T

Baker Creek

Timber
Creek

7.25

Pyramid
Peak
11926'

1.7

Johnson Lake

GREAT BASIN NATIONAL PARK

Snake

Creek

Mt. Washington
11676'

North

Fork

0   1   2 miles

▲ Lincoln Peak
11597'

21 Baker Creek Loop to Baker and Johnson Lakes

RATINGS (1–10)			MILES	ELEVATION GAIN	DAYS	SHUTTLE MILEAGE
Scenery	Solitude	Difficulty				
9	8	7	14	3625	2–3	N/A

AREA Great Basin National Park

MAPS USGS-*Wheeler Peak, Kious Spring*; Earthwalk Press-*Great Basin National Park (1:48,000)*

USUALLY OPEN Late-June to mid-October

BEST July

PERMITS None

CONTACT Great Basin National Park (775) 234-7331

SPECIAL ATTRACTIONS Lakes, scenery, views

PROBLEMS Poor sections of trail

HOW TO GET THERE Along U.S. 50, approximately 58 miles east of Ely, and 90 miles west of Delta, Utah, turn southeast on S.R. 487, following signs for BAKER, GREAT BASIN NATIONAL PARK. After 5 miles, the small community of Baker offers travelers a limited supply of gas, food, lodging, groceries, and auto repairs. In Baker, turn west onto S.R. 488 and drive 5 miles, past the park entrance and the junction with the Wheeler Peak Scenic Drive, to a left-hand turn onto gravel road, signed BAKER CREEK ROAD, TRAILHEAD, CAMPGROUND.

Head south on the well-graded Baker Creek Road, past the campground entrance at 2.9 miles, and continue another 0.5 mile to the loop at the end of the road.

INTRODUCTION Both Baker and Johnson lakes repose majestically in glacial cirques rimmed by rugged walls, beneath the crest of the southern Snake Range. However, these scenic alpine lakes are just two of the many attractions along this trip into the heart of Great Basin National Park backcountry. Baker Creek and South Fork Baker Creek are two delightful streams that tumble down forested canyons as diverse as any drainages in the Great Basin. The verdant, pastoral parkland near the head of the South Fork is particularly stunning.

History buffs will appreciate the area around Johnson Lake, where a long-abandoned tungsten mine has left remnants of a tramway, a stamp mill, and numerous log cabins. Peak baggers will enjoy easy routes to the top of Baker and Pyramid peaks, at 12,298 feet and 11,926 feet the third and fourth highest summits within the park. Hikers with cross-country experience can explore the relatively open terrain away from the trails without much difficulty.

While many of the shorter trails in the more popular area of the Park will see plenty of visitors on a typical summer day, this area affords backpackers a modicum of solitude. Anglers will appreciate the lack of pressure on the resident trout in both the lakes and creeks.

DESCRIPTION Begin hiking along the north bank of Baker Creek near the edge of the transition zone between sagebrush-covered slopes on the right and dense forest of white firs, Douglas firs, and aspens on the left. On a wood-rail bridge you cross a thin rivulet coursing through a meadow and continue to a large grassy flat, where you pass through a cattle gate before reentering the dense forest.

A series of metal signs grabs your attention as you proceed up the trail, markers for a cooperative government snow survey. Continue through cool forest until the path veers away from the creek into the drier vegetation of pinyon pine, mountain mahogany, and sagebrush. This detour is short-lived, as the trail quickly returns to the side of the tumbling stream.

Follow along the creek under shady forest for a considerable distance until you come to a switchback, and then steeper trail, which takes you away from the creek and bends around upstream through mahogany and manzanita. Soon, a scattered, mixed forest of mahogany, white fir, limber pine, and aspen allows filtered views up the canyon. Farther up the trail, the triangular summit of Baker Peak makes an appearance.

You hop over a vigorous side stream near a lovely pool surrounded by lush foliage and wildflowers, a fine grotto suitable for a relaxing break. Continuing up the canyon, ponderosa pine joins a thick mixed forest as you cross a twin-channeled tributary that trickles down rock slabs. Farther on, a wooden walkway bridges boggy meadows, where the steep face of the south canyon wall springs into view.

Pass through a small meadow fed by a meandering rivulet and then head back into mixed forest. After a switchback, cross a side drainage on a four-log bridge and contour back into the main canyon. As you hike along Baker Creek again, pass by a couple of campsites just below a profuse spring, where water gushes over boulders and through a carpet of deep-green grasses and yellow monkey flowers.

Beyond the spring the canyon widens, allowing an expansive meadow to stretch along the far bank. Farther upstream, a series of switchbacks zigzags up the canyon through predominantly Douglas fir forest with a sprinkling of white fir and limber pine. In the midst of the switchbacks is a small campsite next to the creek. Above the last switchback, cross the seasonal outlet from Baker Lake on a four-log bridge and head back to the main channel of Baker Creek. You follow the creek up to Dieshman Cabin, a fairly intact remnant of a bygone era.

Warning: Great Basin National Park contains several old structures like Dieshman Cabin, as well as many other historical artifacts. Please respect these sites, leaving them unmarred for the appreciation of those who come after you.

At the cabin, the trail bends sharply to the right and after some more switchbacks takes you to a junction, 4.25 miles from the trailhead, where a sign nailed to an Englemann spruce reads BAKER LAKE .6, JOHNSON LAKE 1.1.

Continue straight ahead at the junction on a gentle, meandering climb through Englemann spruce forest until the path becomes significantly steeper, near a switchback. You curve around and wander over to the head of the canyon and the rugged cirque holding Baker Lake, 5.25 miles from the trailhead.

Baker Lake, named after an early Snake Valley rancher, is a shallow tarn left over from the last active period of glaciation. In early season, the icy-blue waters of the lake reflect the rugged cliffs rimming the upper walls of the cirque, but by midsummer, the shoreline recedes considerably, exposing a wide band of bleached rock around the diminishing lakeshore. Talus slopes rise up from the water's edge to dark cliffs encircling the lake on three sides. A grassy meadow lined with a dense stand of Englemann spruce on the north shore provides excellent campsites. The shallow lake is home to a reasonably healthy population of trout and the entire shoreline is accessible to anglers.

A mile north of Baker Lake, Baker Peak is the third highest mountain within the Park, after Wheeler and Jeff Davis peaks. A short, technically easy climb ascends the steep slopes above the north side of the lake to the crest of the south ridge, which you then follow to the summit. Across the deep chasm of North Fork Baker Creek are excellent views of both Jeff Davis and Wheeler peaks, as well as the surrounding terrain.

More ambitious mountaineers will welcome the opportunity to double summit by continuing north along the crest to the summit of Wheeler Peak, which at one time was thought the highest mountain in Nevada (Boundary Peak in the White Mountains is 77 feet higher). While an ascent of Wheeler will add extra mileage and elevation to your journey, the climb is straightforward and not technically difficult.

Tip: From Baker Lake, retracing your route back to the junction is not necessary, as a faint path at the southeast shore of the lake makes a more straightforward connection to the main trail. A sign nailed to a spruce reading JOHNSON LAKE 1.4 is near the beginning of the route, and ducks and cairns guide you through the indistinct sections. From the southeast shore, traverse across sloping meadowlands just below talus slides to a boulder field, then continue to the intersection of the main trail, in a broad meadow. A sign attached to an old tree reads BAKER LAKE .3, BAKER LAKE TRAILHEAD 3.7.

Warning: The trail coming up Baker Creek is quite faint, but as you head up the canyon and over the saddle known as Johnson Pass to Johnson Lake, the route is obvious.

Portions of the old trail remain, but the easiest procedure is to ascend the open slopes directly to Johnson Pass. At the 11,294-foot

Johnson Mine

The tungsten ore extracted from the Johnson Mine traveled down to the rock outcropping above the west shore of the lake via the cable that still remains suspended above the slope. From there, mules carried the ore down the canyon to be processed at the mill. After processing, the concentrated ore was transported by wagon to Frisco, Utah, and then sent by rail to a smelter in Salt Lake City. The tungsten operation began just after the turn of the 20th century and continued until the 1930s, when a massive snowslide destroyed the receiving structure on top of the outcrop. Much of the wreckage ended up in the lake and is still visible today near the outlet. The miners attempted to raise the level of the lake by building a rock dam, but the project turned out less than successful.

saddle, the countryside is laid out before you, including Wheeler and Jeff Davis peaks to the north, the continuation of the Snake Range crest to the south, and Johnson Lake directly below. From Johnson Pass, the climb to the summit of Pyramid Peak, at 11,926-foot the fourth highest summit in the Park, is both short and easy, so much so that it would be a real shame to pass up the incredible vista from the top.

More discernible trail leads you away from the pass and across the steep slope above Johnson Lake. At a switchback, a faint use-trail heads up to the remains of the Johnson Mine, where you'll find remnants of an old log cabin, as well as numerous entrances to abandoned mines.

Away from the path to the mine, the main trail continues down the cirque wall, passing directly by the tramway debris on the rock outcropping before reaching the lake basin near the south shore, 1.7 miles from Baker Lake.

Johnson Lake is certainly the most interesting and, in some respects, perhaps the best lake within the Park. The water level at Johnson Lake doesn't fluctuate over the course of the summer like the other lakes in the Park. There are numerous historical artifacts from the old mining days. Steep, dramatic cliffs ring the basin, and rock outcroppings add character to the west shore. A small spring on the limber-pine-dotted hillside above the south shore sends a clear, cold stream of water into the lake. The meandering outlet

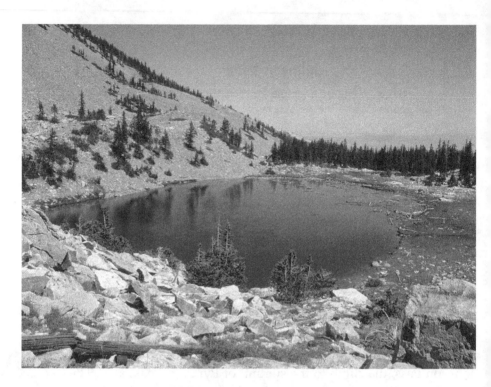

Johnson Lake in Great Basin National Park

courses away from the lake down the canyon through a flower-filled meadow. Campsites can be found on the south shore or beneath the pines near the outlet.

The route from the lake follows the course of an old rocky road alongside the outlet, through spruce forest and past a number of old cabins on a flat just south of the road. Away from the cabins, you continue down the road, following the refreshing outlet until the road crosses over and heads away from the stream. Soon you pass another set of cabins, among which is a large, split-level structure that once housed the stamp mill.

East of the cabins the grade of the old road improves, providing much more pleasant hiking on dirt tread. You leave the spruce behind, and encounter white fir, limber pine, and aspen. Where the trail bends sharply north, a dry campsite occupies a flat. A short distance farther, you encounter a closed Park Service gate. Amid dense forest, 3.1 miles from the lake, you reach a signed junction with the Johnson Lake Trail.

Following directions for SHOSHONE CAMPGROUND, climb steeply northwest up the side of the ridge that separates Snake and Baker creeks, initially through dense aspens before breaking out onto an open sagebrush-covered slope. You reach the crest after 0.6 mile and come to a sign reading SNAKE CREEK DIVIDE, JOHNSON LAKE 1.5. Head directly west along the ridge for a short distance to another sign, where a faint track heads downhill away from the ridge.

A half-mile descent takes you across a couple of seasonal swales and into a broad meadow where the trail disappears. A sign, seemingly in the middle of nowhere, marks a vague junction with the Timber Creek Trail, which is 0.3 mile shorter than the trail along the South Fork, but is not a maintained route. Veer west at the junction and find distinct trail again across the meadow near some trees.

The upper part of South Fork Baker Creek canyon is beautiful parkland with green, sloping hillsides and lush grasses bordering the thin stream. Farther down the canyon, the creek develops a stronger flow, as you cross to the west bank and follow well-graded trail through aspens, white firs, and Douglas-firs.

A large meadow interrupts the forested descent for a while, where the creek adopts a more sedate nature. Beyond the meadow, the grade of descent increases considerably as the creek plummets even more steeply down the lower canyon. A half mile past the meadow, the trail catches up to the rapidly descending creek and crosses to the south side. Eventually, you reach the lower junction with the Timber Creek Trail. After crossing a couple of minor swales and a pair of bridges over Baker Creek, you reach the trailhead, 7.25 miles from Johnson Lake.

POSSIBLE ITINERARY

	Camp	Miles	Elevation Gain
Day 1	Baker Lake	5.0	2650
Day 2	Out	8.95	975

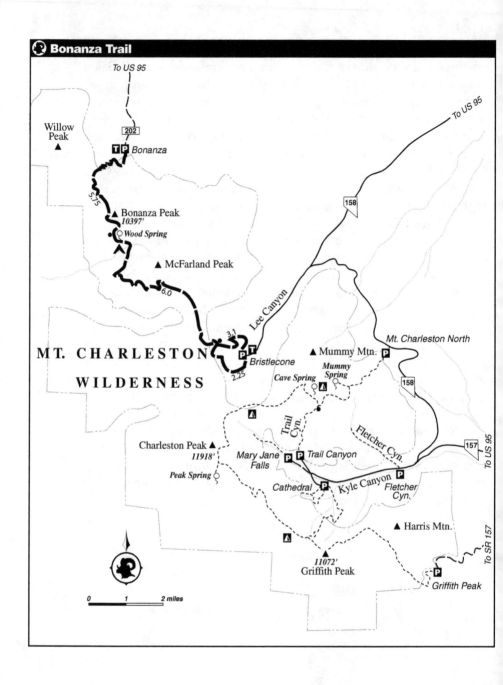

To US 95

Willow
Peak
▲

202

T **P** Bonanza

To US 95

5.75

▲ Bonanza Peak
10397'
○ Wood Spring

158

▲ McFarland Peak

6.0

Lee Canyon

3.1

MT. CHARLESTON

2.25

P **T**

Bristlecone

▲ Mummy Mtn. **P**

Mt. Charleston North

WILDERNESS

Cave Spring

Mummy Spring

158

Charleston Peak ▲
11918'

Mary Jane
Falls

P **P** Trail Canyon

Trail Cyn.

Fletcher Cyn.

157

To US 95

Peak Spring ○

Cathedral

P

Kyle Canyon

P

Fletcher
Cyn.

▲ Harris Mtn.

To SR 157

11072'
Griffith Peak

P

Griffith Peak

0   1   2 miles

22 Bonanza Trail

RATINGS (1–10)			MILES	ELEVATION GAIN	DAYS	SHUTTLE MILEAGE
Scenery	Solitude	Difficulty				
8	8	8	17	5400	2	36

AREA Spring Mountains

MAPS USGS-*Cold Creek, Willow Peak, Wheeler Well, Charleston Peak*

USUALLY OPEN Late May to mid-October

BEST June

PERMITS None

CONTACT Las Vegas Ranger District (702) 873-8800

SPECIAL ATTRACTIONS Views, scenery, bristlecone-pine forest

PROBLEMS Lack of water and campsites

HOW TO GET THERE *START:* Drive north on U.S. 95 to a turnoff signed COLD CANYON, 5.5 miles north of the road to Lee Canyon (State Route 156). Head west for 16.25 miles to a large parking area at the trailhead.

END: There are two choices for ending trailheads in Lee Canyon. You can drive north on U.S. 95 to the junction with Lee Canyon Road (State Route 156) and head west for 14.5 miles to the unsigned turnoff to the trailhead, 100 feet prior to the entrance into McWilliams Campground, then quickly reach the large parking area at the trailhead (Option 1). Or you can continue up the Lee Canyon Road another 0.8 mile to the end of the ski-area parking lot. The unmarked trail begins near the turn-around (Option 2).

INTRODUCTION The Bonanza Trail offers excellent scenery and views of Charleston and McFarland peaks, as well as expansive vistas of the surrounding desert topography. The first 3 miles of trail climb steeply from the toe of the range almost to the summit of Bonanza Peak, traveling through a wide variety of flora that begins in pinyon-pine-juniper woodland, ascends through a mixed forest of white firs, ponderosa pines and limber pines, and culminates near the crest of the range amid bristlecone pines. Much of the middle section closely follows the crest of the Spring Mountains, offering nearly continuous views before a 4-mile descent takes you down to the south trailhead.

One of the most secluded trails in Mt. Charleston Wilderness, this route sees relatively little use, perhaps due to the length and a remote trailhead at the northeast end of the range. If you appreciate solitude, this trail is definitely your best bet in the area.

Warning: Water is scarce—nearly nonexistent except for Wood Spring, 6 miles into the journey. Developed campsites are almost as rare, the most desirable ones being in the bottom of a canyon 0.75 mile below Wood Spring.

DESCRIPTION From the north trailhead, you wander briefly through a clearing to a mixed forest of mahoganies, white firs, ponderosa pines, and pinyon pines, where you begin a long, winding ascent incorporating more than 50 switchbacks and gaining 2300 feet over the course of the first 3 miles. As you climb up the east flank of the range, the forest becomes predominantly white firs, then limber pines, and ultimately bristlecones pines. Views across the desert floor improve with the gain in elevation, as you finally reach the crest of the ridge, 3.1 miles from the trailhead. The vigorous effort required to reach the ridge is rewarded by a view of your progress all the way up from the trailhead, as well as the desert floor some 7000 feet below.

Once you're on the ridge, the grade eases as you follow a more manageable ascent toward Bonanza Peak, passing through exposed outcrops of limestone and scattered bristlecone pines. For the next mile, you ascend mildly along the west side of the ridge to the slope below 10,397-foot Bonanza Peak, where a straightforward, 200-foot, off-trail scramble leads to inspiring views from the summit.

Away from the peak, follow a long descent through bristlecone pines into an unnamed canyon. As you descend, limber pines intermix with the bristlecones, and Charleston Peak makes brief appear-

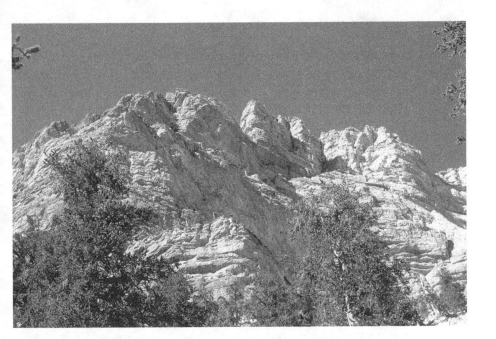

The rugged limestone of McFarland Peak

ances through the trees. Farther down, ponderosa pines start to appear as a series of switchbacks lead to Wood Spring, where a thin pipe transports water straight out of the rock.

Warning: *Make sure you fill all your bottles at Wood Spring, the only reliable water along the entire 17-mile route.*

From the spring, the trail continues a winding descent across dry swales to the bottom of the canyon, at 6.5 miles from the trailhead. White firs and ponderosa pines fill the basin and impressive limestone cliffs form the walls of the upper canyon. A couple of primitive campsites offer the possibility of overnight accommodations, but except for very early in the season when water may be found in the stream, you'll most likely have to get your water from Wood Spring.

Now the hiker is faced with the task of regaining most of the elevation lost in the descent from Bonanza Peak, as a series of switchbacks ascends toward the southwest ridge of McFarland Peak. The 1.25-mile climb culminates in dramatic views of Charleston Peak and the steep limestone cliffs on the south face of McFarland Peak. Once again, you find yourself in the realm of bristlecone pines.

From the crest, follow a gentle traverse past limestone cliffs to the head of the canyon below the precipitous slopes of McFarland Peak. The traverse ends where short switchbacks climb steeply out of the canyon to a low, flat saddle, 10.75 miles from the trailhead. The saddle offers grand views of both McFarland and Charleston peaks.

With the last of the steep ascents behind, you proceed on a mildly undulating 2-mile traverse on or near the ridgecrest, through bristlecone pines with a smattering of limber pines and white firs. Across the deep canyon to the south, Charleston Peak is a nearly constant companion, dominating the surrounding terrain.

At 13.1 miles you encounter an unmarked junction with a path that continues along the ridge for another 0.6 mile before dead ending. Veer east and leave the crest to descend through a dense forest of pines and firs. After three long switchbacks and 0.6 mile, you arrive at a well-signed junction with the Bristlecone Loop Trail in a large gravel clearing, where expansive views include Charleston Peak, Mummy Mountain, and the Lee Canyon Ski Area. From this junction, you have two options for getting to Lee Canyon.

Warning: The Bristlecone Loop Trail is outside of Mt. Charleston Wilderness and is heavily used by mountain bikers. Stay alert, especially on steep downhill sections.

OPTION 1—Head left (east) from the junction and join Scout Canyon Road on a gravel descent that eventually loops around into Scout Canyon. After 1.6 miles, where the road makes a sharp bend to the east near a large grove of aspens, a single-track path descends toward the Old Mill Picnic Area. Remaining on the road, you continue a curving descent and ultimately reach the closed gate above the trailhead, 3.1 miles from the Bristlecone-Bonanza junction.

OPTION 2—Turn right (southwest) at the junction and hike the old roadbed on a gently-rising traverse with good views of the massive limestone cliffs in Lee Canyon. After about 0.25 mile, the road melds into a single-track, mildly graded trail that contours around the head of the canyon through bristlecone-pine forest to the crest of a sub-ridge. Beyond the ridge, a more pronounced descent begins through a mixed forest of bristlecones, white firs, and ponderosa pines. At 1.2 miles from the junction, you reach a seasonal drainage and then follow this swale downslope to an unmarked junction with a path on the left that leads to Gary Abbot Campground.

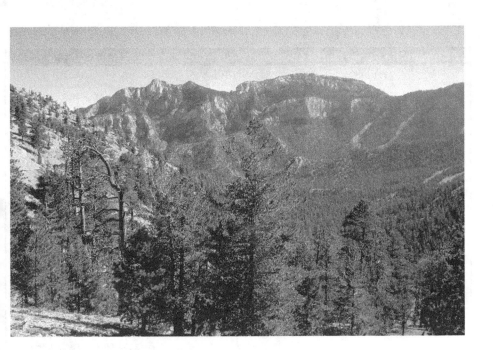

Mummy Mountain from Bonanza Trail

Continue down the vale through white firs and aspens to the open slopes of the Lee Canyon Ski Area, across which is a fine view of Mummy Mountain. Soon you reach the trailhead at the parking lot, 2.25 miles from the Bonanza junction.

POSSIBLE ITINERARY

	Camp	Miles	Elevation Gain
Day 1	Canyon below Wood Spring	6.5	2950
Day 2	Out	10.75	2550

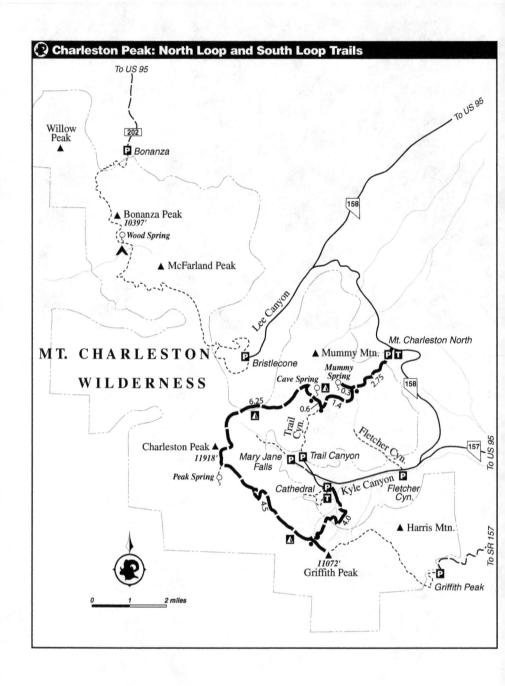

Charleston Peak: North Loop and South Loop Trails

To US 95

Willow
Peak
▲

202

🅿 Bonanza

To US 95

158

▲ Bonanza Peak
10397'

Ⓠ *Wood Spring*

⛺

▲ McFarland Peak

Lee Canyon

MT. CHARLESTON

WILDERNESS

🅿 Bristlecone

Cave Spring

Mt. Charleston North

▲ Mummy Mtn. 🅿Ⓣ

*Mummy
Spring*
Ⓠ

2.75

158

6.25
Ⓐ

0.6

Ⓐ 0.3

1.4

*Trail
Cyn.*

Fletcher Cyn.

157

To US 95

Charleston Peak ▲
11918'

*Mary Jane
Falls*

🅿 🅿 *Trail Canyon*

🅿

Peak Spring Ⓠ

Cathedral 🅿
Ⓣ

Kyle Canyon 🅿

*Fletcher
Cyn.*

4.5

4.0

▲ Harris Mtn.

Ⓐ

11072'
Griffith Peak

To SR 157

🅿
Griffith Peak

0   1   2 miles

23 Charleston Peak
North Loop and
South Loop Trails

RATINGS (1–10)			MILES	ELEVATION GAIN	DAYS	SHUTTLE MILEAGE
Scenery	Solitude	Difficulty				
9	6	9	19.5	5750	2	8.25

AREA Spring Mountains

MAPS USGS - *Angel Peak, Charleston Peak, Griffith Peak*

USUALLY OPEN Mid-June to October

BEST Mid- to late June

PERMITS None

CONTACT Las Vegas Ranger District (702) 873-8800

SPECIAL ATTRACTIONS Views, scenery, bristlecone-pine forest

PROBLEMS Lack of water and campsites

HOW TO GET THERE *START:* Head north from Las Vegas on U.S. 95 to the junction with Kyle Canyon Road (State Route 157) and head west for 17 miles to the junction with Deer Creek Highway (State Route 158). Turn right and follow S.R. 158 past Hilltop Campground for 4.6 miles to the trailhead on the west side of the road at the edge of a wide turnout with room for about a dozen cars.

END: Continue up Kyle Canyon Road (S.R. 157) from the junction with Deer Creek Highway (S.R. 158) for another 3.75 miles to the right-hand turn into the Cathedral Rock Picnic Area. Drive up the access road 0.4 mile, where you'll find fee parking on the left opposite the trailhead.

Warning: *The gate to the picnic area closes at 8 PM in the summer and 6 PM in the fall, so plan on returning to your vehicle before then. If you don't want the hassle of a deadline, or the cost of the parking space, look for parking along the Kyle Canyon Road and walk the 0.4-mile to the trailhead.*

INTRODUCTION An ascent of Charleston Peak is considered to be the ultimate experience in the Spring Mountains by many. The well-engineered and well-maintained 20-mile Mt. Charleston National Recreation Trail, divided into the North Loop and South Loop trails, provides an excellent route to the 11,918-foot summit, which towers over the surrounding terrain by as much as 10,000 feet, offering extraordinary views across southern Nevada, southeastern California, and northwestern Arizona. If not for the insidious pollution from the ever-expanding tentacles of Las Vegas, 300-mile vistas would be commonplace.

Along the way, hikers are treated to additional scenery, including views of Charleston Peak itself and the deep cleft of Kyle Canyon. The route as described below begins from the North Loop trailhead with a steep, nearly 3-mile ascent, followed by a lengthy journey along the crest of the range, and then a steep 4-mile descent to the South Loop trailhead. This is not a true loop trip, however; the two trailheads are separated by 8.25 miles of road.

Tip: *If you're limited to one vehicle, consider an alternate route to Charleston Peak up Trail Canyon, as the trailhead is only 1.4 miles from the South Loop trailhead (see below).*

Despite the arid nature of southern Nevada, the Mt. Charleston National Recreation Trail passes above the pinyon-juniper woodland through a healthy montane forest composed of white firs, ponderosa pines and aspens. Above the montane forest, hikers ramble through limber pines on the way to a vigorous bristlecone-pine forest at the higher elevations, the largest concentration of bristlecones in the state. On the upper slopes of Charleston Peak, summiteers pass above timberline into an alpine-like zone, where only ground-hugging plants can survive the arid, windy conditions. The vegetation within the Spring Mountains is unique, as the range contains nearly forty endemic species, the highest number of any range in the entire Great Basin.

The Spring Mountains are primarily made up of limestone, a porous rock that inhibits anything in the way of perennial streams, but contains numerous caves. Most of the springs, for which the range is named, occur near the base of the range, well away from thirsty hikers. There exists only one permanent source of water directly along the Mt. Charleston Trail, 5 miles from the North Loop trailhead at Cave Spring, where backpackers will find a few humble campsites nearby. After snowmelt, water is absent along the rest of the route, although a couple of springs are accessible from the trail with a minimum of a 0.5-mile detour. Away from Cave Spring, dry campsites with exceptional views will lure overnighters packing sufficient supplies of water.

Warning: Flatlanders will need to acclimatize properly to the altitude of Charleston Peak, and everyone should be prepared to beat a hasty retreat from the upper elevations when thunderstorms are threatening.

DESCRIPTION Leave the parking area on the wide dirt-and-gravel tread of the North Loop Trail and climb through mountain mahoganies and scattered ponderosa pines, crossing the Mt. Charleston Wilderness boundary just after the first of many switchbacks. Farther up the slope, white firs and then bristlecone pines become the dominant conifers. The steep climb brings you to a knob at 1.3 miles, amid a grove of old, gnarled and twisted bristlecone pines that are quite photogenic.

The grade moderates briefly as you pass a dry campsite with excellent views of Mummy Mountain and then resume a steeper climb through mixed forest. A series of twelve switchbacks leads to the top of the bristlecone-pine-covered ridge that divides the Kyle Canyon and Deer Creek drainages. You continue the climb up to a saddle, where you have a commanding view of the massive limestone face at the southern extension of the Mummy Mountain massif, which has a profile suggestive of a 1950s-vintage streamlined locomotive.

Near the top of the ridge, the grade of ascent mercifully eases near a small flat with another dry campsite, and continues a gentle route over to a junction with the trail to Mummy Spring in a saddle below a huge limestone face, 2.75 miles from the highway.

Although taking you 0.6 mile out of the way, the descent to Mummy Spring is well worth the extra time and effort. Lying in a

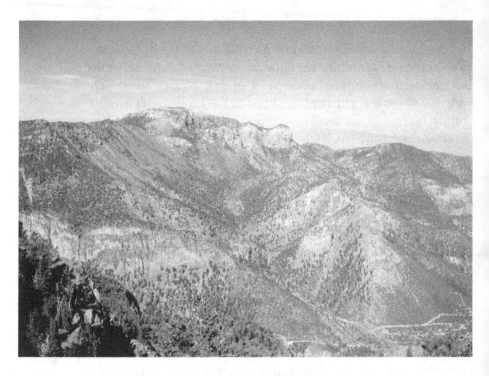

Mummy Mountain from the North Loop Trail

canyon covered with aspens, gooseberries, wildflowers, grasses, ferns, and other lush plants, the northeast-facing ravine creates a cool microclimate well suited to a prolonged rest stop.

For the next 1.4 miles, you follow a curving traverse around the south end of Mummy Mountain to a saddle and a junction with the path down Trail Canyon. A dry campsite is near the junction, with the closest source of water 0.6 mile ahead at Cave Spring.

> **Tip:** *You could shave 2.2 miles of hiking off your trip by beginning at the Trail Canyon trailhead, although the climb is much steeper. To reach the trailhead, drive up the Kyle Canyon Road to a right-hand turn onto Echo Road, 3 miles from the junction with S.R. 158. Follow Echo Road for 0.6 mile to the trailhead near a hairpin turn. The 2-mile trail climbs steeply to the junction. The Trail Canyon option is also favorable for groups with only one car, as the distance between the Trail Canyon and South Loop trailheads is only 1.4 miles.*

From the junction, an initial climb leads through a light forest of predominantly limber pines until you cross an old burn, where young conifers cohabit with aspens and currants. At 4.75 miles from the trailhead, Cave Spring, named for the cave from which it emanates, offers the only water source along the trail for almost the entire trip. Shaded by aspens and bristlecones, the area around the spring offers some primitive campsites, one within the cave itself.

Tip: *Cave Spring is the only opportunity for backpackers to camp near water; however, several dry campsites farther up the trail are more aesthetically appealing.*

The next section of trail ascends the steep slopes below the crest, passing by young aspens and dead snags to some switchbacks. Beyond the switchbacks, an ascending traverse leads past limestone cliffs and through a widely scattered forest of bristlecone and limber pines. More switchbacks take you across rocky slopes below steep bluffs to the ridge crest, where Charleston Peak returns into view across the deep chasm of Kyle Canyon. A rock knoll provides an excellent perch from which to absorb the spectacular views.

Now at the crest, most of the hard work is behind you, as the trail traverses along or near the ridgecrest for the duration of the trip to the slope below Charleston Peak. You continue through widely distributed bristlecone pines and past striking limestone cliffs, passing a number of campsites with extraordinary views along the way. Near the 8-mile mark, you pass the massive limestone cliffs of Devils Thumb before continuing around rugged cliffs and steep slopes to Charleston Peak.

The bristlecone pines left behind, you ascend

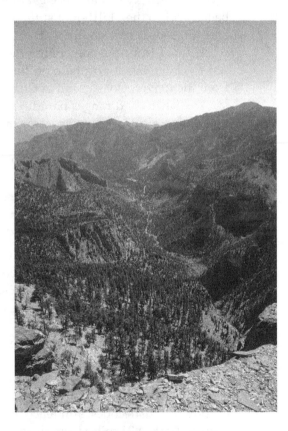

Above Kyle Canyon, North Loop Trail

Griffith Peak, 0.5 mile southeast of the junction, was named for E.W. Griffith, a 19th-century senator who developed the Mt. Charleston area, over 3000 feet below in Kyle Canyon.

long switchbacks that zigzag across the rocky east face of the mountain. Some small tufts of grass and a few tiny plants are all that survive in the rocky soil at this elevation. Finally, four lengthy switchbacks lead to the 11,918-foot summit, where you'll find an antenna and some electronic equipment.

If smog from the burgeoning metropolis of Las Vegas happens not to cloud the atmosphere on the day of your ascent, the views from the long, rocky summit of Charleston Peak are quite spectacular. The basins and ranges parading away from the peak in the distance are almost too numerous to count. Amazingly, Las Vegas and the community of Pahrump to the west, lie nearly 10,000 feet below.

Continuing, you descend from the summit along the South Loop Trail on rocky tread to a traverse just below the crest.

Tip: About 1 mile from the summit, a faint use-trail heads west for 0.5 mile to Peak Spring, a reliable water source that bubbles up from some gravel and runs a short course before disappearing into the soil again.

Away from the junction, follow a mildly ascending traverse for another 0.5 mile, followed by a moderate descent that eventually returns you to the crest, where the superb views down into Kyle Canyon begin. For the next couple of miles, the trail follows the ridge on a mildly descending traverse past limestone cliffs and through bristlecone pines, where you pass a number of fine campsites along the way. Farther down, grassy meadowlands start to cover the ridge, accented by small groves of pines where additional campsites offer the possibility of an overnight haven. Amid a thicker forest of bristlecones, you reach a signed junction with the trail to Griffith Peak, 4.25 miles from the summit of Charleston Peak. Well-used campsites are nearby.

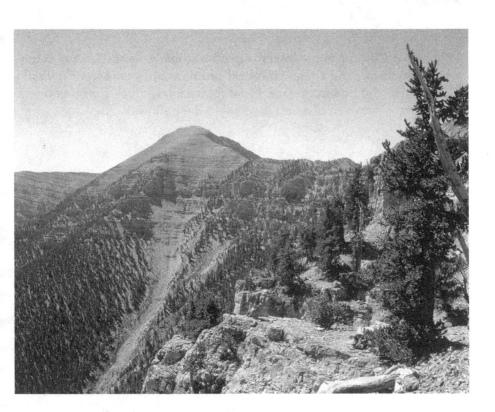

Charleston Peak from the trail, Spring Mountains

> **Tip:** *Hikers with a little extra gas in the tank can make the easy climb of Griffith Peak to add to their list of summits (at 11,072 feet, Griffith is the third highest peak in the Mt. Charleston Wilderness). Follow the Griffith Peak Trail to the south for 0.25 mile, to where a sketchy use-trail branches away to ascend the peak. A short climb past contorted bristlecone pines takes you to the top and a fine 360-degree view.*

From the junction, the South Loop Trail begins the stiff 4-mile drop to the trailhead, over 3000 feet below. Seemingly endless switchbacks take you from the land of the bristlecones into a thick forest of limber pines and then white firs. About 1.5 miles from the junction, you work your way down into the steep-walled lower canyon. Cross the stream channel near a vertical limestone cliff where the stream makes a 50-foot cascade (provided the seasonal stream is flowing). Continuing the stiff descent, pass the wilderness boundary, cross the creek again and reach an old road, where you bend west and cross another branch of the stream. A dense stand of aspen, a plethora of seasonal wildflowers, and the rugged face of

Echo Cliff make the lower canyon a scenic delight. Careful examination of Echo Cliff will reveal multitudinous caves pockmarked across the limestone face. Heading back into thick forest, you hop across a thin rivulet and descend to the trailhead.

POSSIBLE ITINERARY

	Camp	Miles	Elevation Gain
Day 1	7-mile campsite	7.0	2650
Day 2	Out	12.5	2365

Bibliography and Suggested Reading

Carlson, Helen S., *Nevada Place Names*. Reno: University of Nevada Press, 1974.

Charlet, David Alan, *Atlas of Nevada Conifers*. Reno: University of Nevada Press, 1996.

Clark, Jeanne L., *Nevada Wildlife Viewing Guide*. Helena: Falcon Press, 1993.

Cline, Gloria Griffen, *Exploring the Great Basin*. Reno: University of Nevada Press. 1963.

Fiero, Bill, *Geology of the Great Basin*. San Francisco: Sierra Club, 1986.

Hart, John, *Hiking the Great Basin*. San Francisco: Sierra Club, 1991.

Hauserman, Tim, *The Tahoe Rim Trail*. Berkeley: Wilderness Press, 2002.

Kelsey, Michael R., *Hiking and Climbing in Great Basin National Park*. Provo: Kelsey Publishing, 1988

Lanier, Ronald M., *Trees of the Great Basin*. Reno: University of Nevada Press, 1984.

McPhee, John, *Basin and Range*. New York: Farrar, Strauss, Giroux, 1980.

Monzingo, Hugh N., *Shrubs of the Great Basin*. Reno: University of Nevada Press, 1987.

Nicklas, Michael L., *Great Basin: The Story Behind the Scenery*. KC Publications, Inc., 1996.

Stone, Irving, *Men to Match My Mountains*. New York: Berkeley Books, 1982.

Taylor, Ronald J., *Sagebrush Country: A Wildflower Sanctuary*. Missoula: Mountain Press Publishing Co., 1992.

Twain, Mark, *Roughing It*. New York: Penguin Books, 1962.

White, Michael C., *Nevada Wilderness Areas and Great Basin National Park*. Berkeley: Wilderness Press, 1997.

Whitney, Branch, *Hiking Las Vegas: 60 Hikes Within 60 Minutes of the Strip*. Las Vegas: Huntington Press, 2001.

Whitney, Branch, *Hiking Southern Nevada*. Las Vegas: Huntington Press, 2000.

Wuerthner, George, *Nevada Mountain Ranges*. Hong Kong: Nordica International Ltd., 1992.

Zdon, Andy, *Desert Summits: A Climbing and Hiking Guide to California and Southern Nevada*. Bishop: Spotted Dog Press, 2000.

Index

A

animals. *See* fauna
Arc Dome 168, 180
Ash Canyon 47

B

Baker Creek 204–205, 209
Baker Lake 204, 206
Barley Creek 191–192
basin-and-range topography 1
Big Sawmill Creek 166–167
Bonanza Trail 211–215
Brockway Summit 41, 52, 57
Bronco Creek 61, 63, 64, 65
Bucks Canyon 187
Buffalo Creek 81–83

C

Camp Creek 103, 104
Carson Range 15–16
Castle Lake 135, 151
Cave Spring 219, 221
Charleston Peak 218, 222
Christopher's Loop Trail 49
climate 19, 20, 21, 24
clothing (outdoor) 7, 8
Columbine Jeep Trail 180–181
Comstock Lode 15, 45, 48
Cougar Creek 96–97

D

Daggett Pass 39, 42, 43, 44, 45

Danville Pass 192
deer hunting 9
Dollar Lakes 132–133, 152
Duane Bliss Peak 45

E

East Fork Jarbidge River 96, 98–99
East Humboldt Mountains 21–23
Emerald Lake 87, 89–90, 97

F

fauna 17–18, 19–20, 22, 25, 26–27,
   30, 32
Favre Lake 134–135, 150–151
flora 15, 18, 19, 22, 29, 30–31, 32, 33
Furlong Lake 149

G

Galena Creek 62–63
Genoa Peak 44
geology 16, 22, 26, 31, 34
Gods Pocket Peak Trail 101–105
Gray Lake 54–55
grazing 8, 27
Great Basin National Park 32–33
Greys Lake 117
Greys Lake Trail 113–117
Griffith Peak 222, 223

H

Hampton Creek 200
Hendrys Creek 197–198

Hidden Lakes 122
history, human 20–21, 29, 145, 204
horses 11–13

I

Incline Creek 51

J

Jarbidge 87
Jarbidge Lake 87, 89
Jarbidge Mountains 18–21
Jarbidge River 88
Johnson Lake 204,207
Johnson Mine 207
Johnson Pass 206–207

L

Lamoille Lake 133, 152
Liberty Lake 133–134, 151
Liberty Pass 133, 152
Long Canyon 148

M

Marlette Lake 48
Marlette Peak Campground 48
Martis Peak 56
Monitor Range 29–31
Mosquito Creek 192–193
Mt. Fitzgerald 128
Mt. Jefferson 185–187
Mt. Moriah 198
Mt. Rose 59–65
Mummy Spring 219–220

N

North Canyon Campground 46
North Twin River 173–174

O

Ophir Creek Trail 67–73
Overland Creek Basin 145–146
Overland Lake 144, 145, 157
Overland Lake Trail 155–157

P

Paradise Valley 79
Peak Spring 222
permits 8
Pine Creek Trail 184–185, 187
plants. *See* flora

R

rattlesnakes 6
Rebel Creek 77–78
Reese River 164–166
Relay Peak 53
Relay Ridge 53
Right Fork Lamoille Creek 125–129
Robinson Lake 123
Rock Lake 70
Ruby Crest Trail 24, 137–153
Ruby Lakes 131–135
Ruby Mountains 23–25

S

Santa Rosa Range 16–18
Singas Creek 80
Slide Creek 95–96
Slide Mountain 69
Smith Lake 116
Snake Range 31–32
Snow Valley Peak 47
Soldier Creek 120–121
Soldier Lakes 121–122
South Camp Peak 44, 45
South Twin Pasture 163–164
South Twin River 162–164, 174–175
Spring Mountains 34
Spooner Lake 46
Spooner Summit 39, 43, 45, 46
Stewart Creek 179, 181
Summit Trail 75–83
sun 5

T

Table Mountain 190–193
Tahoe Meadows 51–52, 73
Tahoe Rim Trail 39–57

The Table 199, 200
ticks 8
Toiyabe Crest Trail 27–28, 159–169, 179–180
Toiyabe Mountains 25–28
Toquima Range 28–29
Tunnel Creek Road 50
Twin Lakes 50

U

Upper Price Lake 71

W

water 7
Winchell Lake 108, 110
Winchell Lake Trail 107–111
Wines Peak 148, 149
Wiseman Basin 109
Wood Spring 213

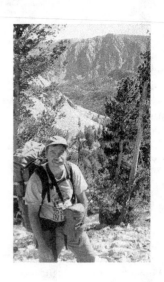

ABOUT THE AUTHOR

Mike was raised in the suburbs of Portland, Oregon in the shadow of Mt. Hood (whenever the Pacific Northwest skies cleared enough to allow such things as shadows). His mother didn't drive, so walking was a way of life for her, as it was for her young son in tow. When Mike reached driving age, he began to explore further afield, hiking, backpacking, and climbing in the Cascades of Oregon and Washington. He further honed his outdoor skills while attending Seattle Pacific University.

After college, Mike relocated to the high desert of Reno, Nevada, where he was drawn to the beautiful and sunny Sierra. This opened the door to many fine adventures, which included hiking forays into the four corners of his adopted state of Nevada.

In the early 1990s, Mike left his last "real" job (with an engineering firm), and began writing full time about the outdoors. His first project for Wilderness Press was an update and expansion of Luther Linkhart's classic guide, *The Trinity Alps*. He then authored *Nevada Wilderness Areas* and *Great Basin National Park*, followed by the *Snowshoe Trails* series and *Top Trails Lake Tahoe*. Mike was also a contributor to *Backpacking California*, and has written articles for *Sunset* and *Backpacker* magazines, and the *Reno Gazette-Journal*.

Mike passes on his accrued outdoor wisdom to students in hiking, backpacking and snowshoeing classes at Truckee Meadows Community College. He continues to live in Reno with his wife, Robin, and their two boys, David and Stephen, along with their yellow lab, Barkley.

Printed in the USA
CPSIA information can be obtained
at www.ICGtesting.com
JSHW031210120923
48167JS00003B/5